Angela G. Gentile

Caring for a Husband with Dementia

The Ultimate Survival Guide

Care to Age Press
Winnipeg, Manitoba
Canada

Caring for a Husband with Dementia: The Ultimate Survival Guide with a Foreword by Marie Marley, PhD.

Email: *caretoage@gmail.com*

Thank you to the following authors for giving permission to use their ideas in this book:

- Chapter 4: Dr. Eric Pfeiffer, for the Seven Stages of Caregiving
- Chapter 5: Dennis T. Jaffe and Cynthia D. Scott for "The Personal Power Grid"
- Chapter 6: Sallie Felton, Life Coach/Transition Specialist, for her list of reasons we don't ask for help
- Chapter 8: Aspen Pub for the symptoms of caregiver stress, written by Linda Alden
- Chapter 11: Dr. Pauline Boss, for use of the concept "ambiguous loss," a term she coined in the late 1970s
- Chapters 12 & 14: Karen Tyrell, for use of the term Therapeutic Reasoning®

Photo Credits:
Front cover: ©Depositphotos.com
Back-cover portrait: Envision Photography
All black-and-white photos: Angela G. Gentile

First Edition
ISBN-13: 978-1505565577
ISBN-10: 150556557X

We wives can handle anything
as long as we know what we're up against.

— Denise, a participant in the Wife Caregivers Project

I dedicate this book to caregiving wives, everywhere.

Acknowledgements

I wish to thank all of the amazing women in the Wife Caregivers Project, the final assignment of my Master of Social Work journey. I designed, implemented, and evaluated a short-term counselling program for caregiving wives of husbands with dementia. I feel honoured to have been part of their lives for a few short months. This book would not have been possible without the invaluable lessons these women taught me.

In addition, I'd like to thank the following people for all of their advice, edit suggestions, and comments that helped me get this book to a finished product I can be proud of: Lynda Greaves, Marie Marley, Ph.D., Karen Tyrell, Dr. Barry Campbell, Frank Kresen and Sue Messruther of Self-Publishing Authors.

I really appreciate all of the support from my mother, Virginia Wilson, and my very good friend, Sheila Roy. Their encouragement and excitement made this journey enjoyable.

Finally, I would like to thank my family for their understanding and patience with me as I went through the writing process: my husband, Agapito; my son, Lorenzo; and my daughter, Simone.

I hope each of you is proud that there is a bit of you in this book. Thank you all from the bottom of my heart.

Angela G. Gentile

Contents

PART THREE
Practical Tips

Foreword

This book focusing on wife caregivers who have a spouse/partner/lover with Alzheimer's disease or a related disorder, is the first book, a one-stop shop for advice and guidance, to deal with this topic. However, although written specifically for wife caregivers, it can apply equally to anyone caring for a loved one with dementia.

The guide deals with a combination of emotional considerations and practical advice. It's a book to be read and then returned to repeatedly for day-to-day guidance in the care of a husband with dementia.

Among the emotional considerations to foster well-being of the caregiver are topics such as caregiver stress, how to ask for help, self-esteem and assertiveness, and moving on after the loss of a loved one. The book is truly the ultimate survival guide, as indicated by the sub-title.

The practical considerations are numerous. There is a long section on how to deal with 25 difficult behaviors. These include – just to mention a few – verbal and physical aggression, bathing, incontinence, sleep problems, sundowning, and sexual expression.

Some other useful topics are covered as well, such as when to consult a physician (of particular importance), long-term care placement, dealing with elder abuse and neglect, and a helpful guide to legal and financial matters.

The guide is also a workbook of sorts. It contains space at the end of each chapter for the caregiver to answer questions related to the information included in that chapter.

First-time author, Angela G. Gentile, MSW, is a clinical social worker specializing in aging. She has more than 25 years of experience working with older adults and their families in a variety of capacities. She has worked in home care, geriatric mental health, long-term care, private practice, health care, and non-profit organizations.

On a personal note, I had seven long years of experience caring for my beloved Romanian life partner of 30 years, who had Alzheimer's. I certainly could have used this guide during my journey. The practical advice would have been great help and comfort to me. I only wish I'd had this book then.

In conclusion, *Caring for a Husband with Dementia,* is a critically important addition to the literature on Alzheimer's caregiving. The pages are chock full of advice that can be directly applied on a daily basis, which will lead to improvements in the care of the loved one and the life of the caregiver.

Marie Marley, PhD
Author, *Come Back Early Today: A Memoir of Love, Alzheimer's and Joy* and co-author, *Finding Joy in Alzheimer's: New Hope for Caregivers.*
March 2015

Introduction

There is something you must always remember.
You are braver than you believe, stronger than you seem,
and smarter than you think.

— Winnie the Pooh

The prevalence of Alzheimer's disease and related disorders is increasing. The rise in age demographics puts more people at risk. Family caregivers all over the world are affected and are struggling with how to manage the difficult task of caring for someone with dementia.

In my last year of Master of Social Work studies in Winnipeg, Manitoba, I was privileged to work with and learn from eight amazing wife caregivers. I developed, implemented, and evaluated a short-term counselling program for the wives, and it was a resounding success. I extend my gratitude to these women, as they shared some of their most difficult and personal stories with me. By sharing what I have learned from working with them, I hope to help other wives (and possibly husbands, other partners, and family members) on their journey of caregiving.

Certain topics resonated with many of the women in the project. Defining dementia, learning about its stages and the stages of caregiving — and about caregiver stress — seemed to be helpful. As one woman remarked, "I have never seen it all laid out like this before."

Knowledge is power, my grandmother always said. Some women found discussing topics such as control, asking for help, supports, financial and legal issues, self-care, self-esteem, assertiveness, and ambiguous loss (when one is physically present but psychologically absent) to be helpful.

Some women were dealing with difficult behaviours. In this book, I have provided tips for managing the 25 most difficult. These tips are intended for the family caregiver, but they may also be helpful to others in both formal and informal caregiving situations. Due to my many years of working with professionals, family members, and those affected by dementia, I felt confident in collating the most helpful and valid tips from various sources. I was also privileged to have Karen Tyrell, Dementia Consultant and Educator, collaborate with me on this topic.

In this book, I describe a new way of communicating with husbands. I use terms such as "Therapeutic Reasoning®" or "therapeutic lying." I ask you to consider dementia as an "external" influence. I include in this book chapters on Long-Term Care and Abuse and Neglect, two of the most difficult topics on the subject, in my opinion.

At the end of each chapter, I provide an exercise: Questions to think about and reflect upon. I encourage you to write down your answers, as this will help guide you in your caregiving journey. You can use the space I have provided, or you can write down your answers in a notebook or journal.

I also encourage you to explore any of the topics I bring up. Search the Internet, or talk to people about what you have learned. Question things. Seek clarity on topics that resonate with you. Clarify things I have just touched the surface of. I wanted to make this book as short and helpful as possible without compromising quality. I have tried to be as accurate as possible, but it is possible I may have made some mistakes along the way. If you do find any errors, please let me know. The errors will be corrected in an upcoming edition. Likewise, if you have any suggestions for improvement, please let me know!

My personal experience of having two grandparents diagnosed with Alzheimer's, combined with my 25-plus years of professional work experience, education, and research has given me much knowledge and insight into aging and how dementia affects our lives. Here are some of the most important concepts I have learned as a clinician:

- People who have dementia rarely can learn or retain new information. They quickly forget.

- People with dementia are not trying to trick or manipulate others. They aren't being purposely annoying, for they are incapable of such a complex task. They simply are trying to communicate their unmet needs. It is our job as caregivers to determine what those needs are.

- People with dementia have a past, and their families are the best sources to describe who they were before their illness. Knowing more about them makes it easier to understand them and provide person-centered care.

- Caregivers are special people. They often overlook their own needs and sometimes require permission to put themselves first. They benefit immensely from talking to others and becoming educated about dementia and caregiving.

- Caregivers have difficulty asking for help.

- As dementia progresses, the difficult behaviour the caregiver has learned to manage may disappear, only to be replaced by another.

- It takes "thinking outside the box" to manage some of the more unique, challenging behaviours.

- Trying new approaches is always recommended, although they might not always work.

- Caregiving has its rewards and challenges. Most people find themselves emerging stronger and more capable from the experience.

- People with dementia are living at home longer than before. There are many reasons people choose not to place their loved ones into long-term care. Whether these reasons are related to finances, preferences, love, obligation, duty, culture, beliefs, or fears, every situation has a unique set of circumstances.

I would like to thank each woman for sharing her story and for trusting me to help on her journey. It was a collaborative approach. I hope the information in this book will be helpful to you. If you wish, please email me (*caretoage@gmail.com*) to let me know your thoughts.

Disclaimer: The information provided in this book is for educational purposes only and is not intended to replace the advice of your doctor, health care provider, financial advisor, or lawyer. You are encouraged to discuss any concerns you have with a qualified professional.

Sincerely,

Angela G. Gentile

PART ONE

Introductory Information About Dementia

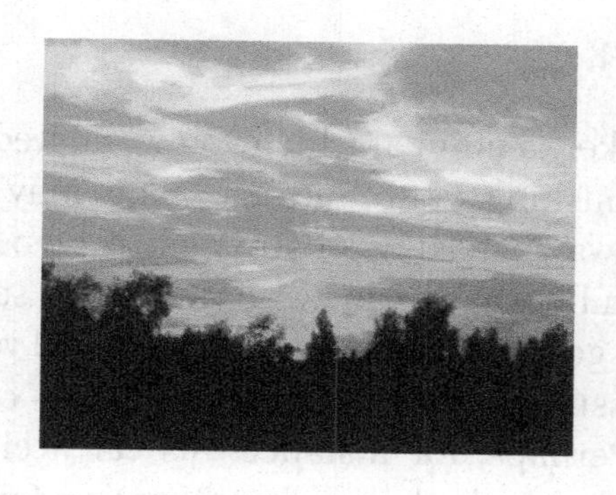

Chapter 1

Knowing Something Isn't Right

From caring comes courage.

— Lao Tzu

Dementia affects many people's lives. The onset of a condition that affects the brain is invisible and often creeps up slowly. In many cases, what starts out as odd behaviour or problems with simple and familiar tasks eventually turns into full-blown dementia. Alternatively, as in the case of a stroke, for example, dementia symptoms can appear suddenly.

As a geriatric clinician and older-adult specialist, I find a lack of services and programs designed to meet the needs of older couples whose lives and marriages are changed and challenged by dementia. My interest in working with older women led me to learn the caregiving wife is a "hidden patient." Thus, I decided to learn more about how I could help women like you in these difficult situations. Although I have been told most of the information I learned can be applied to most caregivers of people with dementia, my primary focus in this book is on you, the wife.

In the Beginning

There was most likely a point at which you wondered if your husband was purposely "pushing your buttons." You may have started to question why he was behaving so strangely. Maybe you thought he was just being stubborn or you were being too sensitive. Perhaps other things were going on in your life that caused you to be on edge. After all, health issues, sleep problems, and stress can cloud the way you see things. Perhaps, for instance, his car accident might have been concerning, but he had a good explanation for why he had run into a parked car. Or when he got lost on his way to the specialist's office, you figured it could have happened to anyone.

Your natural, innate tendency to be a nurturer and caregiver slowly evolved into taking care of more things — and maybe even him — over the last few months or years. You already had raised the children, and you had looked after your ailing mother and his father. Maybe you even were caring for some of the grandchildren. Naturally, your role as a nurturer led you to take on things he needed help with: Reminders to shower or to clean his dentures properly. You might have argued with him at first, but now it's easier just to help.

Many people who develop signs and symptoms of dementia often start by having "senior moments," or temporary memory lapses or difficulty with finding a word. We tend to laugh these instances off, as laughing about our memory problems is more comforting than being concerned. Besides, every person aged 50 or older tends to have occasional senior moments. Many people I have worked with felt, at least at some point, they may have been normal.

This is somewhat like the "how-to-boil-a-frog" phenomenon. If you put a frog into a pot of cool water and then turn the stove's burner on high, the frog won't feel the water come to a boil until it's too late. Dementia is like that. Unless someone has a sudden onset of thinking problems, such as what might accompany a stroke, dementia symptoms often are slow to appear, and they accumulate. The severity might be noticed only when something critical happens.

There Is Something Different About Him

There may be some changes in his personality. For instance, you may notice more arguing. It might be minor at first, and you can become desensitized to it. Before you know it, the arguing and bickering become the norm; you don't make too much of it.

When the kids come around, they might notice something different about Dad. Perhaps he doesn't engage as much as he used to, or he seems a little "off." He might seem more argumentative or forgetful. Not until someone else brings this to your attention do you start to wonder, "What is going on?" You fear it is more than "senior moments." You fear maybe you have a touch of it, too. You may remember his brother has Alzheimer's. Perhaps his mother ended up in a nursing home because of some kind of dementia.

You decide to ask him to go to the doctor for a checkup. He denies anything is wrong. You tell him what you have been observing. He doesn't shave every day like he used to, and now he forgets everything you tell him. He gets angry and annoyed easily. You start to fear there is something else going on with him. You do not want him to lose his driver's license, because that will upset and anger him. Maybe you never got your driver's license. If he cannot drive, how will both of you get around?

You suddenly realize maybe it *isn't* you; maybe there *is* something wrong with him. You have trouble denying the facts. He used to be able to pay all the bills, but you have had to take on this task because he was mixing things up. He never used to be so agitated and argumentative; his personality has changed. After 40 or 50 years of marriage, you have never seen him like this.

It might take a serious matter for you to realize the magnitude of the problem. For instance, when he had not returned by suppertime after visiting a friend and picking up milk, you worried and called the police. They found him safe but disoriented.

Dementia can come in many forms. According to the Alzheimer Society of Canada (2014),

> The word *dementia* is a general term that refers to many different diseases. Different types of dementia are caused by different physical changes to the brain. Some dementias are reversible, meaning they can be treated and cured. Some are irreversible, meaning there is no cure yet.

10 Warning Signs of Alzheimer's Disease

Alzheimer's disease is the leading cause of dementia. The Alzheimer Society of Canada (2014) gives these signs:

1. **Memory loss that affects daily functioning.** A person with Alzheimer's disease may have problems remembering recent things.

2. **Familiar tasks become difficult.** For example, people who have prepared meals all their lives might find the task challenging.

3. **Problems with language and communicating become apparent.** Trouble finding the words — or substituting words — is common for someone with Alzheimer's disease.

4. **Disorientation to time and place.** For example, a person with Alzheimer's disease could become lost on his own street, or he might forget what year it is.

5. **Poor or decreased judgement.** A person with Alzheimer's disease might refuse to see a doctor for a medical problem, or he might wear layers of clothing on a hot day.

6. **Abstract thinking skills become impaired**. A person with Alzheimer's disease might not know what the numbers in a cheque book mean, for example.

7. **Misplacing things.** A person with Alzheimer's disease might put things in odd places, such as an iron in the freezer or a wristwatch in the sugar bowl.

8. **Changes in mood or behaviour.** A person with Alzheimer's disease might experience mood swings and go from happy, to sad, to angry, without apparent reason.

9. **Changes in personality.** A person with Alzheimer's disease might become confused, suspicious, or withdrawn and act out of character.

10. **Loss of initiative.** A person with Alzheimer's disease might become passive and require cues and prompting to take action or to get involved.

Although these warning signs are specific to Alzheimer's disease, it is not uncommon to see many of these symptoms in other types of conditions that cause dementia. Dementia is defined as a syndrome or a condition that affects the way the brain functions. It is often of a progressive or chronic nature. Some of the more common conditions associated with dementia are Alzheimer's disease and other progressive neurocognitive disorders, Parkinson's disease, stroke, Huntington's disease, Multiple Sclerosis, and vascular disorders (such as multi-infarct dementia). There will be more information regarding dementia in Chapter 3.

Dementia, Delirium, and Depression

There are three conditions that may overlap and look similar in older people: dementia, delirium, and depression. Depression is also a condition that needs to be considered when someone is experiencing memory problems. Sometimes one condition can make the other(s) worse, and you can have one, two or all three. Thus, it is important a qualified health care professional provides a thorough assessment.

Delirium is a medical emergency in older people and can result in death. The onset of this confused, delirious state is often sudden. A physical problem, such as an infection or the effects of medication, could be the cause.

He/she may have periods of lucidity (alertness), as the symptoms often fluctuate. It is often caused by a physical problem such as an infection, or it can be caused by the effects of medications. Many other factors can cause delirium, such as unmanaged pain. It is important to know delirium is a reversible condition.

For example, a person who is given a prescription of eye drops could suddenly become confused, lack concentration, and start hallucinating. Likewise, a person with a systemic infection, such as caused by a bladder infection, also could become delirious. There are many causes of delirium, and people who have had a bout of it are susceptible to recurrences. A delirious older person is too often misdiagnosed as having a progressive form of dementia, so the key is to have a thorough assessment by a qualified and experienced professional. This will be discussed further in Chapter 2.

Exercise:

I realized there was something seriously wrong when:

____

____

____

What I did about it was:

____

____

____

I am feeling:

____

____

____

References:

Alzheimer Society of Canada (2014). *Dementias*. Retrieved from: *http://www.alzheimer.ca/en/About-dementia/Dementias*

Alzheimer Society of Canada (2014). *10 Warning Signs*. Retrieved from: *http://www.alzheimer.ca/en/About-dementia/Alzheimer-s-disease/10-warning-signs*

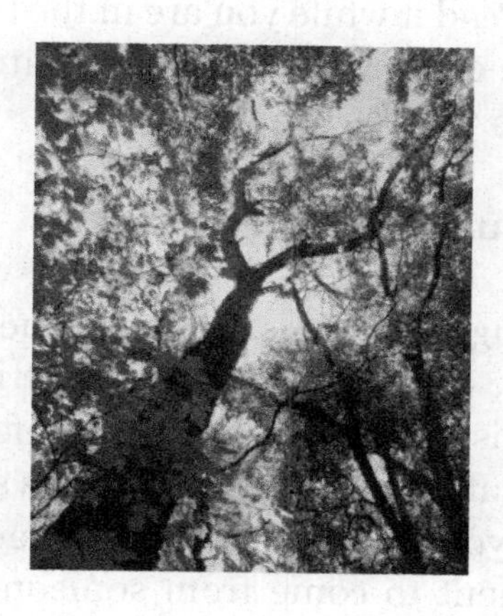

Chapter 2

Getting a Diagnosis

Doctors diagnose, nurses heal, and caregivers make sense of it all.

— Brett H. Lewis

Suddenly you realize something isn't right — there is a real problem — and you no longer can avoid it. Or you can't bear to believe something is wrong and you may need help. It's been going on far too long — for months or even years. With the support of a close family member or friend, you decide to have your husband assessed by a doctor to find out what may be going on.

Once you realize there is a real problem, it is scary to think it may be serious. The best way to handle the situation is to start by bringing your husband to the doctor. Go in with him to the appointment. Some doctors won't allow you to be present for the appointment and will require legal papers to prove you have authority (more on this in Chapter 16). Document any sensitive information you may not want to share aloud in front of your husband. The doctor can look at the information later or read it while you are in the office. You also could send the notes to the doctor before the appointment so he or she is aware of the concerns.

Diagnosing the Cause of Dementia

The process of figuring out what is causing dementia is often not that simple. For instance, the family doctor might not feel comfortable making the diagnosis. Some doctors will refer to a geriatrician, neurologist or psychiatrist. Some psychologists specialize in working with older adults. If your husband is 65 or older, it would be a good idea for the assessment to come from someone who specializes in conditions affecting older adults, such as a geriatrician.

The doctor will likely order or administer cognitive tests, blood tests (including liver function), a urinalysis, and maybe even a chest X-ray to rule out pneumonia. There may be a referral to a geriatric psychiatrist, a geriatric mental health clinician, or a team of professionals. Other medical problems must be ruled out before there can be a definitive diagnosis. In some cases, the process can take a few months. It can cause you to worry and make you feel like you are on an emotional roller coaster.

You might suggest to your husband it has been a long time since his last complete physical, so you want him to have one. It is important to get blood work, a urinalysis, and some kind of neuro-imaging of the brain. Common types of blood work for cognitive or memory problems include hemoglobin, red blood cell count, white blood cell count, sodium, fasting blood sugar, HgbA1C, urea, creatinine, serum albumin, serum calcium, thyroid-stimulating hormone (TSH), and vitamin B12 (cobalamin).

A computerized tomography scan (CT) or magnetic resonance imaging (MRI) scan of the brain is recommended. The CT scan may be infused, which means injected with a contrast dye to enhance the images. A positron emission tomography (PET scan) may be ordered.

Some of the common symptoms of dementia can be eliminated once their reasons are determined and treated. Medical tests can help rule out any other medical problems or insufficiencies that may be contributing to decreased cognitive functioning. For example, someone with a bladder infection may appear confused, but antibiotic treatment could clear the confusion as well as the infection. There could also be a delirium component involved if there are other medical problems or conditions that can result in decreased or impaired brain functioning.

Mental or memory tests also will help with the diagnosis. I am most familiar with the Mini-Mental State Examination (MMSE) and the Montreal Cognitive Assessment (MoCA). There may be other tests available in the future, but these are the commonly used ones as I write this. Both of these tests have a total score of 30. The MoCA is a more sensitive test and is difficult for some people. It is possible someone with dementia can score high on the MMSE and low on the MoCA, so it is always helpful to do the MoCA when the MMSE score is higher (25 or more).

Other common tests include the clock-drawing test and the months of the year in reverse order. In the clock-drawing test, which is also included in the MoCA, a person must draw a large circle and put the numbers of a clock in it. Then the person is asked to draw hands to display 11:10. The way he/she draws the clock and its hands helps the assessor determine how well he/she can reason, problem solve, and access working memory. When a person is asked to list the months of the year in reverse order, the assessor quickly and easily can determine his/her concentration and memory skills.

Many different tests can be performed. None of the tests alone determines a diagnosis of dementia. The test results can help determine if your husband is having difficulties in his thinking skills. This will naturally prompt other tests and assessments to help determine a diagnosis.

Treating Dementia

Once a diagnosis is made, your husband's doctor will most likely discuss treatment options. The type and severity of the dementia-related condition will determine which treatment will be prescribed. For example, Lewy Body Dementia does not respond well to certain types of medications. There are commonly known medications prescribed for Alzheimer's disease. There is no known cure for dementia, however. Medications are prescribed to help manage or lessen some of the symptoms, and they don't work for everybody. There are always new treatments being made available, so ask the doctor about options for your husband's condition.

Assessing Abilities in Daily Living Activities

The other important aspect of diagnosis is assessing how your husband is able to manage or handle day-to-day tasks. For example, if your husband is no longer driving, can no longer pay the bills, and is having trouble remembering to take his medications, his daily living or functioning is affected. If you notice he is having trouble with simple things such as knowing what day it is, or if he has abandoned his hobbies, he may have dementia. Difficulties with problem solving and word retrieval also are key symptoms you should mention to the doctor.

Consider your husband's ability to stay safe. For example, help him if he forgets to take his medications or turn off the stove.

Learning About Dementia and Sharing the News

Once a diagnosis is made, your husband's doctor will most likely share this information with you. It is a good idea to name someone else, usually a close family member, as a backup in case you are unavailable to discuss your husband's condition with the doctor. Be sure the doctor knows who this person is and has the necessary contact information. Some doctors will require legal proof that you are authorized to deal with your husband's health-related matters, and, as I mentioned previously, this will be discussed in more detail in Chapter 16.

The next step is to become educated on dementia so you can be prepared for what is to come. You may feel a sense of loss and sadness. You might worry about your future and whether you can handle it. We will focus more on grief and loss in Chapter 11.

After becoming educated about the condition, you must decide with whom to share the information. Your children, his siblings, other relatives, his friends, and the grandchildren need to know about his condition in order for them to understand him and his behaviour. Their knowing about your husband's condition will help them support you. Encourage them to learn about dementia as well, so that they can interact with him in an appropriate and respectful manner. Check out some of the great resources available through your local Alzheimer Society or Alzheimer's Association. In addition, the next chapter will provide you with more information.

Exercise:

The tests my husband has had are:

____

____

____

My husband needs extra help with:

____

____

____

With regard to the diagnosis, I feel:

____

____

____

These people know about my husband's condition or need to know:

____

____

____

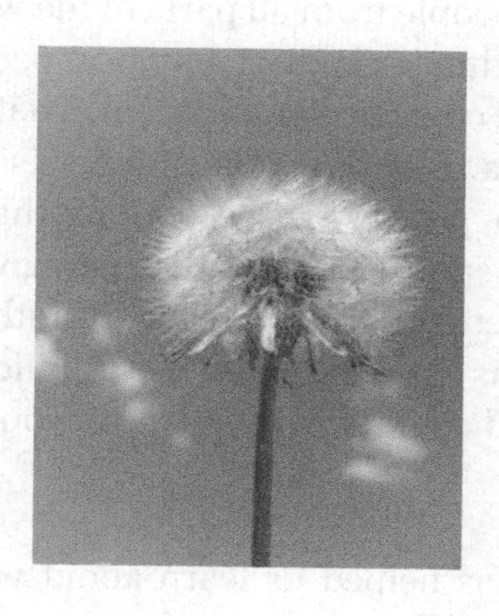

Chapter 3

Understanding Dementia

When people say, "You have Alzheimer's," you have no idea what Alzheimer's is. You know it's not good. You know there's no light at the end of the tunnel. That's the only way you can go. But you really don't know anything about it. And you don't know what to expect.

— Nancy Reagan

The risk for getting dementia (also known as neurocognitive disorders) increases with age. It is not normal to develop dementia, however. In *Rising Tide: The Impact of Dementia on Canadian Society,* a 2010 report published by the Alzheimer Society of Canada, one in 11 Canadians older than 65 currently lives with dementia. In fact, one in three Canadians older than 80 is living with dementia. In other words, if there are three couples who are older than 80, two of those six people likely could have dementia. The older you become, the greater the likelihood that there are many other couples who share your situation.

Dementia affects people from all parts of the world. In Canada, the Alzheimer Society estimates in 2011, 747,000 people were living with dementia or a related cognitive impairment. That's almost 15% of the population in Canada. By 2031, that number is expected to double, affecting 1.4 million people. If we add to that all of the family members, including spouses, plus other caregivers, that is a lot of people touched by dementia. Worldwide, if nothing else changes by the year 2050, there is expected to be 115.4 million people living with dementia or a related cognitive disorder. As you can imagine, this is a global concern.

Modern science has helped us learn about what it means to live healthy lives, and our life expectancy has increased due to lifestyle changes and technological advances. Longer lives, however, do not necessarily mean healthier lives. We still are at risk for developing chronic illnesses, such as dementia-related conditions. Therefore, the longer we live, the higher our chances for developing dementia. (However, it's important to note that not all conditions of cognitive impairment are chronic and progressive and can sometimes be reversed. See Chapter 2 for more details.)

Alzheimer's Disease Facts and Figures, a 2014 report from the Alzheimer's Association, states a woman aged 65 has a one-in-six risk of developing dementia; the risk is one in 11 for men. The difference is accounted for by women's longer life expectancy.

Defining Dementia

Dementia is a worldwide problem. The World Health Organization's *Fact Sheet on Dementia* (2012) describes dementia as the following:

> "Dementia is a syndrome – usually of a chronic or progressive nature – in which there is deterioration in cognitive function (i.e., the ability to process thought) beyond what might be expected from normal aging. It affects memory, thinking, orientation, comprehension, calculation, learning capacity, language, and judgement. Consciousness is not affected. The

impairment in cognitive function is commonly accompanied, and occasionally preceded, by deterioration in emotional control, social behaviour, or motivation.

A variety of injuries and diseases, such as Alzheimer's disease or stroke, primarily or secondarily affect the brain and can cause dementia.

It is one of the major causes of disability and dependency among older people worldwide. Dementia is overwhelming not only for the people who have it but also for their caregivers and families. There often is a lack of awareness and understanding of dementia, resulting in stigmatization and barriers to diagnosis and care. The impact of dementia on caregivers, families, and societies can be physical, psychological, social, and economic."

Dementia is a term used to describe many symptoms associated with a decline in memory or other thinking skills that impair a person's ability to perform daily tasks and activities. Some compare dementia, as a deteriorating condition of the brain, with how arthritis affects the joints. The dementia-affected brain also has been referred to as an injured or damaged brain, as noted in the popular book, *The 36-Hour Day,* by Mace and Rabins.

Dementia and Related Disorders

Dementia is present in all parts of the world. According to research done in the United Kingdom, 62% of people with dementia have a diagnosis of Alzheimer's disease. 17% of people have Vascular Dementia (including stroke), and 10% have a mixed form of dementia (such as Alzheimer's disease and Vascular Dementia occurring together).

Figure 1: Prevalence of Dementia in United Kingdom (source: *alzheimers.org.uk*, 2014)

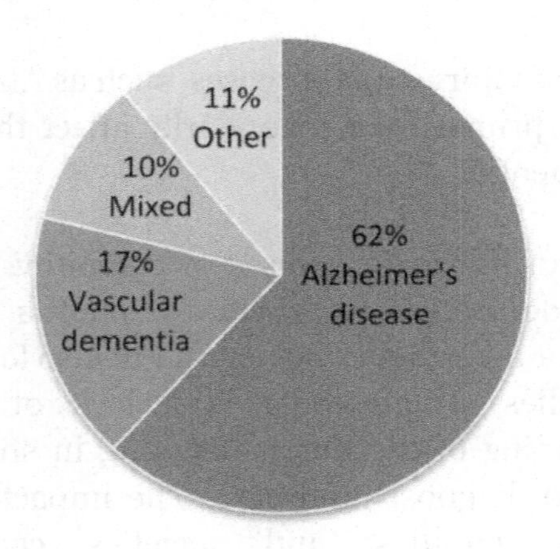

In terms of "Other," the following breakdown is given:

- 4% Lewy body dementia
- 2% Frontotemporal dementia
- 2% Parkinson's disease dementia

The remaining 3% includes:

- Huntington's disease
- Traumatic brain injury
- Creutzfeldt-Jakob disease
- Wernicke-Korsakoff syndrome
- Down syndrome
- and others

Alzheimer's disease is the leading cause of dementia in the world. The World Health Organization states 60 to 70 percent all dementia cases may be caused by Alzheimer's disease. It is not uncommon for people to say "dementia" when they are actually talking about Alzheimer's disease. But as you can see from the statistics above, not all dementia is due to Alzheimer's. That is why it is important to understand the cause of dementia in order to treat it. Currently there is no known cure for any of the above-noted conditions.

Stages of Dementia

Dementia and caregiving both have stages that are helpful to know about. The stages of caregiving are described in the next chapter. The Global Deterioration Scale (also called the Reisberg Scale) describes seven stages of cognitive decline, which is typically seen in the course of a progressive condition like Alzheimer's disease. These stages can help you, the caregiver, understand where your husband is at in terms of the progression of his condition. In Alzheimer's disease, decline usually takes a slow and progressive course. People with Alzheimer's disease tend to lose about two points on the Mini-Mental State Examination per year. Stage progression might not proceed fluidly; he might seem to go in and out of stages, with each successive stage emerging with time. Not all forms of dementia progress in the same way.

Your husband may be in the earlier stages of Alzheimer's disease, which are identified with minor forgetfulness, and he may be having more difficulty managing his usual hobbies. As his disease progresses through the stages, things become more difficult for him. His memory loss could include forgetting parts of his own family history, or he may forget who you are. You most likely are familiar to him, but he may think you are his mother or sister.

The Global Deterioration Scale is presented here for you as a reference guide to help you get an understanding of a progressive form of dementia. In Vascular Dementia, there is a similar but different course, which I will explain later.

The Global Deterioration Scale (*www.alzheimer.ca*):

1. **No Cognitive Impairment**. The person functions normally.

2. **Very Mild Cognitive Impairment**. Dementia is not present, but the person may experience memory lapses and problems with remembering familiar words.

3. **Mild Cognitive Decline**. Dementia is still not present, but other people may start to notice the person experiencing some difficulties with short-term memory, finding words, or performing tasks. Health care professionals can detect problems upon cognitive testing.

4. **Moderate Cognitive Decline**. This is also known as early-stage dementia. The person may start to demonstrate more noticeable short-term memory problems and have trouble with mathematics or organizing complex tasks. Mood fluctuations are more noticeable. He or she may no longer be able to drive safely.

5. **Moderately Severe Cognitive Decline**. Dementia is now at a middle stage. There are very noticeable gaps in memory, and people in this stage may become confused as to their location or the date. They might forget where they live or what school they had attended. They might require help choosing appropriate clothing for the weather or season. They still can manage eating and toileting on their own.

6. **Severe Cognitive Decline**. Dementia in the middle stage continues to worsen. Personality changes and inability to manage daily living tasks independently become more challenging. The person may no longer be able to go to the toilet on his own, as he may forget to flush or wipe properly. He may have trouble voiding in appropriate places, or he may soil himself. He may remember his own name, but he could have trouble remembering who family members are. He may require assistance with dressing and, if not provided with help, may put clothing on improperly or put shoes on the wrong feet. Sleeping patterns may become mixed up. He may demonstrate major behavioural problems or may wander off and become lost.

7. **Very Severe Cognitive Decline**. In late-stage dementia, individuals lose the ability to respond to and communicate with those in their environment. Conversations will be difficult or impossible. Movement is not controlled, and they will require help with almost all activities, including eating and using the toilet. Abnormal reflexes cause difficulty for the caregivers, and muscles grow rigid. Difficulty with chewing and/or swallowing can increase the risk for choking.

Health care practitioners also can stage the dementia another way, through what is called the "Clinical Dementia Rating" scale (Norris, 1993). Dementia can be rated as very mild, mild, moderate, or severe, depending on level of functioning in the following areas: Memory, orientation, judgement and problem solving, community affairs, hobbies, and personal care. Knowing the stage of the disease can help you understand and prepare for what is to come.

It is also common to see Alzheimer's disease categorized into four stages. According to the Alzheimer Society of Canada, these four stages are: Early, Middle, Late, and End of Life. Their website breaks down these four categories quite well and applies a "palliative approach" to care at the end of life. It is similar to the kind of approach that would be applied to someone who is at the end stage of terminal cancer, for example.

Vascular Dementia

All of the wives in the Wife Caregiver Project were caring for husbands who had Vascular Dementia (also known as Multi-Infarct Dementia). Vascular Dementia has been found to be the second leading form of dementia after Alzheimer's disease, accounting for approximately 20% of all cases of dementia (Alzheimer's Society of Canada, 2014). When considering a condition like Vascular Dementia, it is important to note it is usually because of a stroke or a series of mini-strokes. Brain cells are deprived of oxygen and die. Different parts of the brain are affected, which makes every presentation different. Some parts of the brain are left relatively unaffected. Diagnosing Vascular Dementia can be difficult, and sometimes it is accompanied with Alzheimer's disease, which is termed a "Mixed Form of Dementia."

Vascular Dementia often progresses in a "stepped" manner. Think of it like going down stairs, versus down a ramp. Each stroke or attack on the brain results in more loss of functioning (doing) or cognitive (thinking) skills. Symptoms may worsen and then remain unchanged for a long period, perhaps months or years. Fluctuations in abilities and mood may be seen on a daily basis. It is possible, if a person never experiences another stroke, symptoms may not worsen over time.

Many people with Vascular Dementia retain their personality and more normal levels of emotional responsiveness until the later stages of the disease. They can present well in a group of people, which makes it hard for others to really understand or believe a problem exists. The person with Vascular Dementia may be aware of his problems, making him prone to depression.

Each person's experience with dementia will be different. In many cases, the person's death will result from a stroke or a heart attack due to their high cardiovascular risk factors. Preventing or lowering these risks is highly recommended. Discuss this with a health care professional for ways to help prevent further decline.

Exercise:

In terms of stages, I think my husband is in stage __ because:

____

____

____

What I fear most is:

____

____

____

References:

Alzheimer Association (2014). *2014 Alzheimer's Disease Facts and Figures*. Retrieved from *http://www.alz.org/downloads/Facts_Figures_2014.pdf*

Alzheimer's Association (2014). The Seven Stages of Dementia. Retrieved from *http://www.alz.org/alzheimers_disease_stages_of_alzheimers.asp*

Alzheimer Society of Canada. *Dementia Numbers in Canada*. Retrieved from *http://www.alzheimer.ca/en/About-dementia/What-is-dementia/Dementia-numbers*

Alzheimer Society of Canada (2010). *Rising Tide: The Impact of Dementia on Canadian Society*. Retrieved from *http://www.alzheimer.ca/~/media/Files/national/Advocacy/ASC_Rising_Tide_Full_Report_e.pdf*

Alzheimer Society of Canada. *Stages of Alzheimer's disease*. Retrieved from *http://www.alzheimer.ca/en/About-dementia/Alzheimer-s-disease/Stages-of-Alzheimer-s-disease*

Alzheimer Society of Canada. *Vascular Dementia*. Retrieved from *http://www.alzheimer.ca/en/About-dementia/Dementias/Vascular-Dementia*

Alzheimer Society UK. *Dementia 2014 Infographic Text Only Version*. Retrieved from *http://alzheimers.org.uk/site/scripts/documents_info.php?documentID=2761.*

Morris, J. C. (1993). The clinical dementia rating (CDR): Current version and scoring rules. *Neurology*, 43(11), 2412-2414.

World Health Organization (2012). *Dementia Fact Sheet No. 362*. Retrieved from *http://www.who.int/mediacentre/factsheets/fs362/en/*

PART TWO

Emotional Considerations

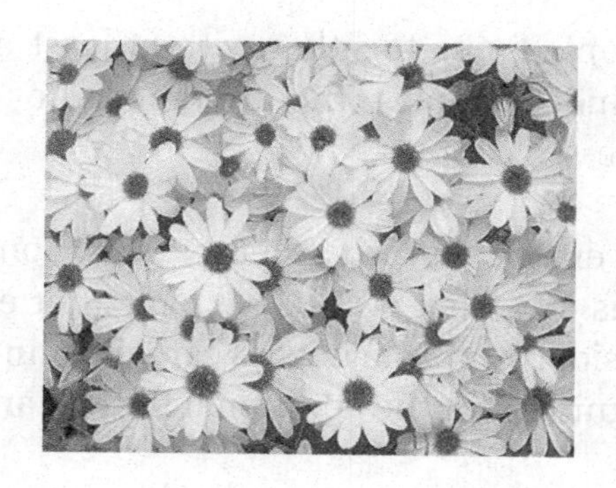

Chapter 4

Understanding Caregiving

Alzheimer's caregivers are heroes.

— Leeza Gibbons

In a report issued by Statistics Canada (2012) titled, "Portrait of Caregivers," we learn that most caregivers in Canada spend about three hours weekly assisting others. These include friends, neighbours, parents, and other family members (not their children). Children spend about 10 hours weekly helping their parents, which is quite high.

What was most interesting is spouses score highest, reporting an average of 14 hours weekly assisting and caring for their ailing partners. It is also noted this number may be lower than it actually is because the tasks of caregiving may be seen as an extension of the role as spouse.

According to Statistics Canada, in 2012, the number of senior couple families had increased by 17% over the previous four years. It is estimated in 2015 there are more than 2,000,000 older couples living together, and this number is growing. These "couple families" consist of two people living together with at least one person older than 65. This includes couples who are married or common-law. It also includes same-sex couples.

You may not even see yourself as a caregiver. Some women I have talked to say, "It is just what we do. We look after each other." I am asking you to consider your role now as caregiver, in addition to wife. You deserve recognition for the additional burden and challenges put upon you.

In terms of your role as caregiver, you are not alone. According to the Alzheimer Society of Canada, one in five Canadians older than 45 provides care to older adults living with some form of long-term health problem. Of those who are family members, a quarter of them (200,000) are 75 or older, according to 2008 statistics. Unfortunately, caregiving can take its toll both physically and psychologically. The World Alzheimer Report (2012) states approximately 75% of caregivers will develop psychological problems.

These statistics alone are enough to highlight the importance of individual proactive measures, including educating yourself on the topic of dementia and taking care of yourself and your husband in the best way possible.

Understanding how the caregiving role affects you emotionally and learning what you will need at different stages will also help you prepare for this important and commendable role.

Stages of Caregiving

Much like your husband will go through stages of dementia, you will experience stages of caregiving. The Seven Stages of Caregiving I like to refer to and teach to caregivers is based on the work of Dr. Eric Pfeiffer, MD (1999). In his practice as a doctor, he has worked with many caregivers and people with dementia. He has described a way to explain the stages of caregiving. These stages are very closely tied to the Seven Stages of Dementia (see previous chapter). As you read about these stages, see if you can identify with any of the feelings or situations. Pay attention to how you feel as you read through the list. Some of the women who have learned about these stages say they have "never seen it all laid out like this before." It helps them see where they have been, where they are at, and where they are headed. It can help you prepare, both practically and emotionally.

You will see terms like "Long-Term Care," "Institutions," "Residential Care Facilities," "Personal Care Homes," and "Nursing Homes" to describe a place where your husband can live and be cared for. These types of accommodations provide 24-hour care and supervision provided by teams of health care aides, nurses, and other health care professionals. Meals, medications, recreational activities, and other programming and services are provided in most of these places. Some accommodations offer specialized dementia care units or other special-needs options. I will generally shorten it to "Home" or "Homes" for sake of brevity.

In this section, I ask you to try to *focus on yourself*. For many wife caregivers I work with, I have noticed it is very difficult for them to separate themselves as an individual person from their husbands. Your life for the past few months or years has most likely revolved around your husband. Now is the time to focus on you — your feelings and how your situation affects you.

The Seven Stages of Caregiving (Pfeiffer, 1999):

1. **Dealing with the Impact of a Diagnosis**. When it is realized something is seriously wrong and a diagnosis of dementia is made, it is a life-changing event. Feelings of sadness, fear, and ambiguous loss (he is physically there but psychologically absent) can cause close family members to feel overwhelmed. They may feel a sense of loss and grief over what could have been. This is the beginning of the caregiving journey.

2. **Making the Decision to Be a Caregiver.** When a loved one has a diagnosis of dementia, a decision needs to be made to either have someone else look after the person or to take on the responsibility yourself. In the case of an adult child and parent, there are sometimes other children who can share the responsibility. In the case of a spouse, it is often "expected," or the well spouse feels "obligated" to look after their ailing partner. Whether it is to prevent burdening other family members or is done out of love and caring concern for the person with dementia, a decision is made to move forward as caregiver.

3. **The Long Journey of Caregiving at Home**. When a family member is in the early, middle, and later stages of dementia, there are different needs that the primary caregiver must consider. Refer back to The Seven Stages of Dementia, and you will see that the demands placed on the caregiver increase as the dementia symptoms progress. Outside help may be needed to provide respite or some other aspects of care. Other family members or friends can be asked to help more. Special approaches to deal with behavioural issues that arise may be required. Safety issues may become more of a concern. The caregiver needs to be mindful of her own needs in order to keep herself healthy and to develop effective coping skills. (The concept of Coping with Difficult Behaviours and how to manage them will be discussed more fully in Chapter 14.)

4. **When It Is Time for Long-Term Care Placement.** It is highly likely that a difficult decision will have to be made at some point. Some people choose to have their loved one moved to an institution such as a Nursing Home or Residential Care Facility. Sometimes the situation escalates to the point where hospitalization is necessary. Depending on how serious the situation is, some will have the decision made for them by doctors or other health care professionals. The issues surrounding this topic are often complicated and difficult for the caregiver, and sometimes the person living with dementia resists the idea. Reasons for placement may very well include that the caregiver is

burnt out, unwell, or can no longer provide safe and adequate care. Sometimes the health of the person living with dementia is deteriorating, and the complexity of the situation is too much for the caregiver to handle.

5. **Providing Caregiving to an Institutionalized Loved One.** Caregiving does not end when a loved one moves into a care facility. The role changes to providing oversight of the care provided and visiting the loved one.

6. **When Your Loved One Dies.** Grief and relief are experienced. Although the death was to be expected, it still comes as quite a shock. The loss and grief you feel are normal. Although you have most likely experienced ambiguous loss and anticipatory grief, this is a permanent loss. Give yourself time to process. You may also experience feelings of relief. You may be relieved that your husband is no longer suffering, no longer discomforted. Even though you may feel relief, at the same time, you may feel unwarranted guilt. (Loss will be discussed in more detail in Chapter 11.)

7. **Resuming Your Life after Caregiving.** Many caregivers emerge feeling more capable and stronger after the caregiving experience. Some choose to take on the cause of helping others who are going through a similar experience. Others move on to new and different experiences.

The Caregiving Wife

I know that you, as a wife of a husband with dementia, have a different set of circumstances than, say, a daughter who looks after her mother. You have (or had) an intimate relationship with this person, and you made vows to this person which included looking after him "in sickness and in health." The unique and intimate relationship between a husband and wife is very different from all other relationships. For example, the adult child looking after his or her parent or a sibling looking after a brother or sister does not have the same level of relationship as that found in a marriage. A live-in spouse caregiver has a different type of relationship, and this is why I wrote this book.

The wives I worked with stated their role as wife changed as their husband's dementia progressed. Almost all of the wives said their sex life was nonexistent. The marital relationship changed when dementia started to affect their husbands' behaviour. For example, one wife said her husband is no longer an equal partner in the relationship, and now she has to do everything. Another woman said she feels like she is "looking after a toddler who gets up in the night." Most of the women stated they considered their husbands as a "dependent" now. He was no longer able to care for himself, and she became the caretaker, much like a mother looks after a child.

In my observation with the wives, I have learned it is helpful for a wife to help her husband focus on what he is still capable of, versus taking on an overbearingly "motherly" role. Focusing on his strengths (versus his weaknesses) provides a better chance of making him feel better about himself, resulting in a happier husband. It is very easy for a wife to take over simple tasks he can do himself. For example, instead of gathering up his laundry, ask him to do it. You may have to ask him a couple of times, but if he is able to get the job done and you are able to praise him, this will result in positive feelings all round. Or, you may want to ask him to sweep the floor. Pick something he can do that will make him feel useful and appreciated. Try searching the Internet for "101 things Alzheimer's"; you will find a long list of ideas to choose from.

The connection to your lover, although at times it may have been (or still is) tumultuous, may be strong. The very fact you are reading this now indicates you are committed to going all the way – "until death do us part." The other sad thing to know here is dementia tends to hasten death, especially in the case of Lewy Body Dementia. In Vascular Dementia or a Mixed Dementia, often a stroke takes the person's life. The increased cardiovascular risk factors cause an increased risk of heart attack or stroke. In Alzheimer's disease, it is often the inability to chew or swallow, or a decrease in the desire to eat that causes problems resulting in death. Pneumonia is a common cause for death in those with dementia.

Caregivers and Depression

I also want to bring to your attention the issue of depression. In a study done by Mausbach *et al.* in 2013 involving Alzheimer's disease, 125 caregiving spouses were interviewed and compared with 60 non-caregiving spouses. The researchers found 40% of those who were caring for a spouse with dementia had depression, versus only 5% of those who did not have a spouse with dementia. I would like you to keep this important finding in mind, as you may, at some point, feel depressed.

The signs of depression (according to the *Diagnostic and Statistical Manual of Mental Disorders, 5th Edition*) include depressed mood or increased irritability, decreased interest or pleasure, significant weight change or change in appetite, change in sleep patterns, change in activity, increased fatigue or loss of energy, feelings of guilt or worthlessness, difficulty concentrating, and suicidal thoughts. These changes can affect your social life or daily functioning and coping. If you feel you may be depressed, please discuss with your doctor for treatment options.

Caregiver stress and burnout can affect people in different ways. There is a risk in "caring too much" and "trying to do it all." In Chapter 8, we will talk more about these issues and how they can be prevented.

The Positive Side of Caregiving

Many people who provide care to loved ones have positive things to say about caregiving. Those who are able to see the benefits of caregiving experience lower levels of depression. In a study done by Haley *et al.* (2003), the following benefits of caregiving were identified by caregivers:

- A sense of giving back to someone who has cared for them
- A sense of knowing a loved one is getting excellent care
- Personal growth
- Increased meaning and purpose in one's life

You may want to add some of your own ideas of what you see as a positive benefit of caregiving. Maybe it's because it makes more sense financially to have you and your husband living together. You may feel good because you are upholding your marital vows. You will have an opportunity to reflect on this in the exercise below.

If you asked me, I would describe the caregiving wives I have met as kind, courageous, selfless, tolerant, and committed. They are humble, above all else. You may identify with some or all of these traits. Think of more traits unique to you that you can add.

To close this chapter, I want to share, as Dr. Pfeiffer (1999) has found, the dementia caregiver often emerges stronger and more capable than before the caregiving experience.

Exercise:

In terms of the stages of caregiving, I think I am in stage _____ because:

____

____

____

What I dislike most about caregiving is:

____

____

____

What I like most about caregiving is:

____

____

____

Some of the benefits of caregiving for me are:

____

____

____

References:

Alzheimer Society of Canada. *Dementia Numbers in Canada*. Retrieved 18 Jan 2015. *http://www.alzheimer.ca/en/About-dementia/What-is-dementia/Dementia-numbers*

Haley, W. E., LaMonde, L. A., Han, B., Burton, A. M., Schonwetter, R. (2003). "Predictors of Depression and Life Satisfaction Among Spousal Caregivers in Hospice: Application of a Stress Process Model." *Journal of Palliative Medicine*, 6, 215-224.

Mausbach, B. T., Chattillion, E. A., Roepke, S. K., Patterson, T. L., and Grant, I. (2013). "A Comparison of Psychosocial Outcomes in Elderly Alzheimer Caregivers and Noncaregivers." *American Journal of Geriatric Psychiatry*, 21 (1), 5.13.

Pfeiffer, E. (1999). Stages of Caregiving. *American Journal of Alzheimer's Disease and Other Dementias*, 14:125.

Sinha, Maire. (2012). Portrait of Caregivers, 2012. Statistics Canada. Retrieved from *http://www.ccc-ccan.ca/media.php?mid=378*

Statistics Canada. Table 111-0034 – *Seniors' characteristics, by family type, age of oldest individual and source of income, annual (dollars unless otherwise noted)*, CANSIM (database). Retrieved from *http://www5.statcan.gc.ca/cansim/a26?lang=eng&retrLang=eng&id=1110034&tabMode=dataTable&srchLan=-1&p1=-1&p2=35*

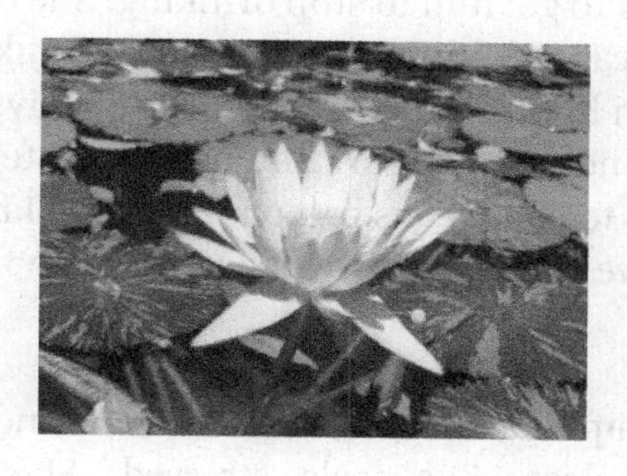

Chapter 5

Personal Power Grid

God grant me the serenity to accept the things I cannot change, courage to change the things that I can, and the wisdom to know the difference.

— Reinhold Niebuhr

This chapter is all about learning how to know when you can take control of a situation and when you should let it go. It is about learning how to choose to react to a situation in a way that is healthy and helpful. I am reminded of The Serenity Prayer as noted above.

One of the most difficult things for most people to do is to recognize when it is time to let go of something. I am referring to when we are in a difficult situation, and we want to change it. Our natural tendency is to want to take control of a situation in order to relieve pain and suffering. We want to prevent problems, and we think we know what is best. Our years of experience in this world and our increased wisdom sometimes become our own worst enemy.

For example, if Jane's husband is an alcoholic, she may try doing everything she can to get him to stop drinking. She can monitor all of his activities, she can ask him how much he is drinking, and she can beg and plead with him to stop drinking. Ultimately, none of this will change her husband's behaviour. She is so invested in his life, she thinks it is her job to change his behaviour. What Jane does not want to accept or believe is she cannot change him. He has to want to do that for himself.

Jane is caught up in a situation where she has no control, but she continues nonetheless. She feels stressed. She is engaging in "ceaseless striving." Imagine spinning your wheels in the mud. It is a waste of your time and energy. The healthier option for her would be to accept he is an alcoholic, let him know that, if and when he is ready to make a change, she will be there for him, and to "let go" of the control.

Most of us need to feel in control of our lives. The problem is when we have no control over a situation, and we try to make a change by getting involved. We mean well, and we try to influence or control a situation by doing certain things and taking action. A lot of our time can be invested in a situation we have no control over. This is like banging our heads against a wall. We tend to lose sight of the things we have control over, and we fail to let go of things we have no control over.

The other side of not being able to control a situation is the ability to *master* it. These are situations where we have the ability to take control of a situation, and we choose to take action. For example, if I want to lose weight, and I know I can do it by eating less and exercising more, I could "master" the situation by doing just that. We can master any situation where we have ultimate control and we take action. Sometimes we may fail at it, but at least we are attempting to be successful at something.

Alternatively, we may have control over something, but we fail to take action. This is where we choose to ignore a situation or simply "give up." This can be perceived as being neglectful as well.

Mastering and Letting Go

To help you understand this concept, I would like to share with you The Personal Power Grid (Jaffe & Scott, 1984, 1988). This is a visual representation of a way to describe the concept of control (see Diagram 1). The grid can be divided into four quadrants. On top are Mastery and Ceaseless Striving, and on the bottom are Giving Up and Letting Go.

The two most healthy options in most cases are having Mastery (have control and take action) and Letting Go (have no control and take no action). Letting go can be hard to do, and it takes a lot of courage to accept things the way they are. Learning to accept or let go of something you do not like and cannot change can be so freeing.

Ceaseless Striving and Giving Up are both unhealthy ways of dealing with stressors that can result in feelings of stress, depression, low self-esteem, and frustration. Over time, these problems can cause us physical and mental health problems. It can cause conflict in our relationships. It can create barriers to our own peace and contentment.

Diagram 1. The Personal Power Grid

Personal Power Grid	Have Control of Outcome:	Have No Control of Outcome:
Take Action:	**Mastery**	***Ceaseless Striving***
Take No Action:	***Giving Up***	**Letting Go**

When it comes to using the Personal Power Grid in your life as caregiver, as you come across challenges and conflict, it would be a good idea to reflect on this Personal Power Grid and to see where the problem fits within this framework. Ask yourself these questions: Do you have control over what is happening? Is there any way you can influence the situation? What would it take to change the situation? If the answers are "No," then it may be best to let it go, versus endless tries and repeated failed attempts. Alternatively, what are you struggling with that can be "Mastered" or "Let Go"?

For example, if your husband continuously rearranges the dishes in the cupboards after you tell him you like the way the dishes are arranged, it may be best for you to "let it go." You cannot change his compulsion to move the dishes due to the dementia. You realize this activity is keeping him busy, and he is not at risk of harm by doing so. Letting go will help you come to peace with this situation.

On the other hand, if your husband wants to go for a walk, and you feel he is at risk of getting lost, you can arrange to have someone go with him. You have control of the outcome by keeping him safe, and you take action to "master" the situation. It is a win-win situation. He gets to go for a walk, and you are able to keep him safe by having your neighbour take him out. You choose to take action, and you have control of the outcome.

As you begin to apply the principles of the Personal Power Grid, you may start to feel less stress in your life. A big part of reducing the stress in our lives includes asking others for help. We will talk more about this subject in the next chapter.

Exercise:

These are the things I have control over:

____

____

____

These are the things I do not have control over:

____

____

____

Something I would like to Master is:

____

____

____

Something I would like to Let Go of is:

____

____

____

Reference:

Jaffe, D. and Scott, C. (1988), *Take This Job and Love It: How to Change Your Work Without Changing Your Job*, p. 161. Simon & Schuster.

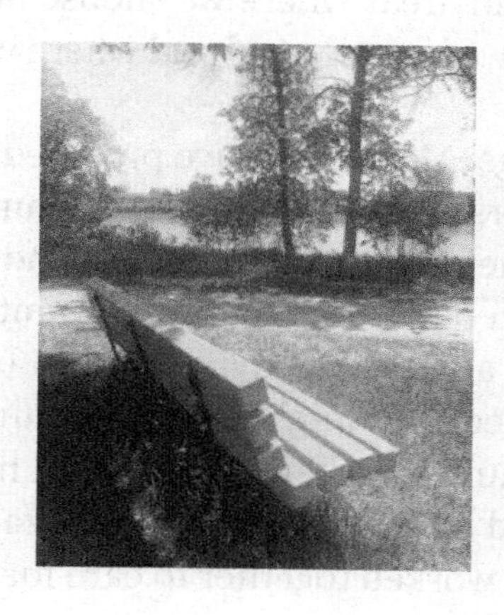

Chapter 6

Asking for Help

Sometimes asking for help is the most meaningful example of self-reliance.

— Unknown

A very important part of self-care is recognizing when it is time to ask others for help. This is especially true for caregivers. Most of us strive to maintain independence and prefer to have control over our lives. Some of us were brought up believing that asking for help is a sign of weakness. Admitting you can't do something on your own can cause you to feel like you are dependent and a failure. You are not a failure. The kind of attitude that can get a caregiver into trouble is when you think, "No one can do as good a job as me." Being able to ask for help when you need it is an important part of being proactive.

If we refer back to the Personal Power Grid mentioned in the last chapter, we see there are areas of our lives where we have control of the outcome — and areas where we don't. There are also areas where we choose to act — and areas where we choose not to act. Asking for help is an area where we have control and where we can choose to act.

We are social beings. Most of us have provided care and some kind of assistance to others at various points in our lives. We have no trouble agreeing to help someone if asked, and we often feel good about doing so. It is in our human nature to want to help. As women, we tend to value the ability to provide care to others more so than men. It is an innate need, we might say, something we are born with. It goes back to the hunter-gatherer way of life many years ago. The men would go out and hunt while the women stayed behind with the children. The women worked together to care for the community and tend to their kin.

Realizing You Need Help

When you become a caregiver of a spouse with dementia, you may soon realize you can't do everything on your own. Maybe your own health is beginning to fail, and you are not as physically capable of doing things as you used to be. Arthritis may set into your shoulders, and now you realize you can't reach those things on the top shelf. Your husband can't help you, either, because of his failing condition.

You need to make a choice at this point. Do you go without those items on the top shelf, or do you ask someone to help you get those items down? The way I see it is you are not losing your sense of independence by asking someone to help you with this task. You are, in effect, mastering the situation by taking action. You have the ability to make your life more manageable if you just ask for a little help.

In other cases — those in which more than a little help is needed — it may take more courage to ask for what is required. For example, you may want to go on a weeklong trip to see a relative who lives hours away, and you know you can't leave your husband alone. He won't go into a facility for respite, so you feel trapped. In this case, you will most likely benefit from asking a family member, such as a son or daughter, to stay with him. The asking part is the hardest.

What do you have to lose? If your family member is not available, at least you asked. If your family member is available, and it works out, you can rest assured that your husband is well looked after and safe. You will be able to go on your trip, and you will get your much-needed change and getaway. If you don't go on that trip, you may start to resent your husband and question what kind of life you have.

Reasons We Don't Ask for Help

Sallie Felton, Life Coach/Transition Specialist, has compiled a list of reasons we don't ask for help, even though we know we need it. I have taken her list and adapted it to what a wife caregiver may be saying to herself. See if you identify with any of these reasons.

- I don't want to burden anyone. He's my husband; he's my problem. They didn't ask for this.

- If I ask for help, I am being selfish. It is not okay to ask for help.

- I will feel obligated to help them in return, and I don't have time or energy for that.

- I am not that important. They never ask me how I am doing, so they won't care.

- I don't want people to know how bad it is. I don't want them to know about his dementia. They won't believe me, anyway.

- I feel they have better things to do than to help me. They are too busy with their own family and commitments.

- I don't want to come across as someone who cannot handle X, Y, Z... I am a strong and independent person. I have been that way all my life.

- I don't want to appear weak. Weakness is a sign of failure.

- I don't want to be perceived as someone who is "failing." He is my husband, and I took a vow to look after him – so I must.

- I don't have the time to look for help. I am too busy doing everything around the house, and I have the responsibility to look after both of us. I have to get him to all his appointments. That's all I can handle right now.

- He won't let anyone else come into the house. He doesn't see the need for supervision, and I don't want to upset him.

- No one else can look after him as well as I can.

I have noticed one of the most common reasons caregivers are reluctant to ask for help is they believe they are the best person to provide care to their spouse. They believe no one else can do it better than they can. Even though this may be true, it doesn't mean other people can't provide adequate and, in the case of family, loving, care. It may be a humbling experience to ask for help, but, with some practice, you will get better at it.

There are many reasons women find it difficult to ask for help. I have talked to wife caregivers who have said that, although it is hard, you *just have to ask for help*. You get used to it. In many cases, you will be pleasantly surprised at how eager people are to help you.

Everyone's reasons for not asking for help will be different. Maybe you can add more reasons to the list above. Reflect on your reasons in the exercise at the end of this chapter.

How to Ask for Help

Once you decide you are going to ask for help, the difficulty may lie in *how* you ask for help. It is important not to make the request sound weak, such as, "I was wondering if you *might* like to stay with Dad on Sunday while I go out to get my hair done and have lunch with my friend. *It's just a thought.*" It's better to be affirmative and confident in your request. You may want to say instead, "If you are free on Saturday, *I hope you can stay* with Dad while I go out for a bit. I want to get my hair done and have lunch with Mary."

Consider the task that needs to be done, and think of someone who is good at it or likes to do it. For example, if your neighbour likes to help you shovel snow or cut your grass once in a while, ask him if he could help you out a little more. Ask your daughter who lives nearby to pick up some groceries for you the next time she's out. Make it easy for them. Offer some choices of things that you think they may be interested in helping out with. Matching the task to the person will help make it easier for everyone.

When you ask for help, be sure you are clear about what you want. Clarity helps prevent disappointment and sets up the helper for success. Make sure the person understands why you want the help. For example, you could say, "I am under a lot of pressure right now, and, if you could find out more about that tax credit for me, I would feel a lot better." (More about tax credits in Chapter 16).

If you meet with resistance or a refusal, just consider that maybe it is not a good time for the person. You may want to suggest that he or she just think about it. Maybe next time, it will work out better, so don't be afraid to ask again. However, if people say that they are already overwhelmed with their own responsibilities, respect this, and seek out someone else who has more free time and is able to help.

If asking for help is new to you, you may want to start by asking for small things first. Taking baby steps towards bigger "asks" can help you learn what works and what doesn't. See who is more willing and available to help you. Take it slow at first. Asking a neighbour to pick up milk for you is less of a big deal than asking your son to stay with your husband for a weekend while you go away on a trip to see your sister.

As your situation changes and you find ways other people and organizations can help, you will most likely see the benefits of having a "team" to join you on this journey. Your team could consist of family, friends, professionals, or community services. Joining a Caregiver Support Group through your local Alzheimer Society is also a way that you can connect with others. You can learn about how to ask for help and find out what kind of help is available.

The Mayo Clinic (*www.mayoclinic.org*) has a great website that I often refer to. They have an article called "Alzheimer's Caregiving: How to Ask for Help," written by Mayo Clinic Staff. You may want to do an Internet search for this article and check it out.

Caregiving Alone Can Be Stressful

One of the dangers of not asking for help is becoming stressed with all of the demands of caregiving. Over time, you may find that there are more and more things that need to be done. It can become overwhelming. If you don't ask for help in the earlier stages, the stress may slowly creep up on you. Remember the analogy, "How to boil a frog"? I have also asked caregivers, "What will happen to your husband if you are no longer able to provide care for him?"

Some caregivers are in denial, and they don't even realize that they need help. The stress can creep up on them, and, all of a sudden, they are surprised by how stressed out they are. I worked with one wife who was saying how great things were going. It appeared to be a situation she was handling quite well. Then, one day, I called her to confirm our appointment together, only to find out that she had suffered a stroke. She admitted it was too much for her to handle, and the stress had finally gotten to her. Stress can become a silent killer. She was lucky, but not everyone is.

Consider seeking help as a sign of personal strength. Knowing what your limits are and warding off caregiver stress and burden in both the physical and emotional senses are key concepts in terms of maintaining your own sense of personal well-being. You will be a better wife and caregiver for it.

It is important to look after yourself first. This concept is the same as what we learn in air travel safety instructions: *Put your own oxygen mask on first*. As women, as caregivers, we need to make sure we are looking after ourselves first so that we can look after others. Self-care will be discussed more in Chapter 8. In the next chapter, we will explore what types of help are available.

Exercise:

The reasons I have difficulty asking for help are:

____

____

____

In terms of asking for help, I have learned:

____

____

____

What would be a small request I could make, and who could I ask?

____

____

____

Reference:

Felton, Sallie (2013). Why do we not ask for help? *Positively Positive*. Retrieved from *http://www.positivelypositive.com/2013/03/07/why-do-we-not-ask-for-help/*

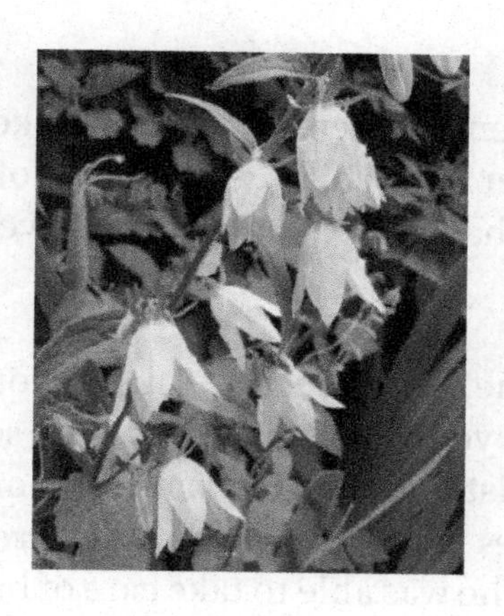

Chapter 7

Practical and Emotional Support

You can do anything, but not everything.

— David Allen, Productivity Consultant

You do not have to go it alone. In our society, caregivers (like you) of people living with dementia are valued members. Our society has realized the value and importance of helping to enhance the caregiver experience. In order for caregivers to do a good job, they require support — emotional as well as practical — education, and resources from the people around them.

In most cases, you will be considered the primary caregiver, and there will be a secondary caregiver, such as an adult child, who will be there for you as a backup. Wife caregivers, like you, are in a more difficult situation because they are "expected" to take care of their husbands. It is not only our own expectations we put on ourselves but also the expectations of society. Most women do not even give it much thought when they take on the role as primary caregiver to their husbands.

It is much like when you were expected to take care of others. You may have looked after your children or your mother or father as she or he aged. You may have cared for other relatives or friends over the years.

However, this time, it's different. This is your life partner. This person is the love of your life. Maybe you had some difficulties, but you chose to go the distance. The intimate relationship and emotional bond you share makes your relationship as a caregiver different. This man is your partner; he was able to take care of business. He was your protector and provider. He is father to your children. Now, your roles have changed. You have to take on more and more. The responsibilities and tasks have crept up on you, and now you realize you are feeling stressed.

Not only do you have to take care of most things around the house, now you have to take care of him as well. He has become a dependent. You can no longer rely on him to pay the bills or drive you to your appointments. You can't do it all, and you know that, if you don't find some help, you will crumble.

Seeking Outside Support

There are many resources available to you. Once you make the decision to seek assistance, you need to know where to turn. Your children or friends might be telling you that they know of some resources or programs that you may want to consider. Here is a rundown of the main sources of support (both practical and emotional):

- **Family and Friends**. This is the most obvious and accessible resource for most people. The difficulty here is asking for help. Some people are fortunate to have family and friends who just offer help, without having to be asked. But there are other people with whom we need to be more clear about what our needs are, and we need to be more assertive in our requests. Adult children, especially daughters, are the most helpful and involved, according to research. If you do not have a daughter, a daughter-in-law may also be just as helpful. Don't be afraid to ask your son or your son-in-law to help. Your husband's siblings may also be able or willing to assist. Neighbours can also be lifesavers in a pinch.

- **Government Programs and Services**. In some jurisdictions, such as in Canada, there are provincially funded programs that provide practical supports. For example, a Home Care assessment by a social worker or nurse can help determine what supports are needed. They can advise you about what other resources are available in your area. Some examples of the kinds of help you may be able to access are bathing assistance, respite (both in-home and in-facility admissions), Adult Day Programs, and dressing or grooming assistance.

- **The Alzheimer Society of Canada**. There are many opportunities for education and support through the local chapter of the Alzheimer Society. They also have support groups and a phone line (1-800-616-8816 in Canada) which you can access. The programs are available to anyone caring for people whose conditions range from mild cognitive impairment to late stages of dementia. *www.alzheimer.ca*. In the USA, call the Alzheimer's Association, 1-800-272-3900.

- **Your Husband's Doctor**. Letting the doctor know the difficulties you are encountering can help the doctor understand what the problems are at home. He or she may order more tests, a referral to a specialist, or a referral to Home Care or another similar program.

- **Paid Caregivers**. There are many private businesses and home care companies who provide health care aides and companion services for a fee. Some services offer to do errands for you. You can even hire someone to do your housekeeping, if needed.

Private-duty nurses are also available. There are even moving companies who will pack for you. Ask your friends or family for a referral. Alternatively, check your local yellow pages listing or the Internet for services near you.

- **Canadian Red Cross – Community Health Services**. In some parts of Canada, the Red Cross Society offers the following: Community Support Services, Health Equipment Loans, Home Care, and Community Initiatives. Check out the Canadian Red Cross Society website at *www.redcross.ca* for contact information in your area.

- **Private Therapist**. I have found in my practice that many women rely on their adult children for emotional support. They often feel that it is not appropriate to be sharing their "family problems" with strangers. However, it may be difficult for a son or daughter to help you because they may have their own issues or may be too busy to help or to listen. You may not want to burden your friends or neighbours with your concerns. Therefore, sometimes it is helpful to talk to a person who is neutral to the situation and has the expertise to help you see things from a different perspective. A private therapist, such as a social worker or psychologist who has experience working with older adults and families, would be a great choice. Your doctor or local Alzheimer Society may be able to recommend someone to you.

- **Private Dementia Consultant.** This is a fairly new concept. A Dementia Consultant is a professional who can support you one on one to address your questions and concerns. She/he can work with you to address difficult behaviours and offer you emotional support. Search the Internet for a "dementia consultant" or "dementia practitioner" near you. Their popularity is on the rise.

There are many ways you can get help and support for what you are going through. In order to take care of yourself and your husband, you may have to rely on others to assist you. Consider them part of the "team." If your husband were in a Home, there would be a team of caregivers and professionals looking after him there. Give yourself permission to ask for help. It is an investment in your well-being, because stress can take its toll over time. Know what your limits are, and take care of yourself.

Exercise:

I could use help in the following areas:

____

____

____

I will contact the following people or agencies for some help:

____

____

____

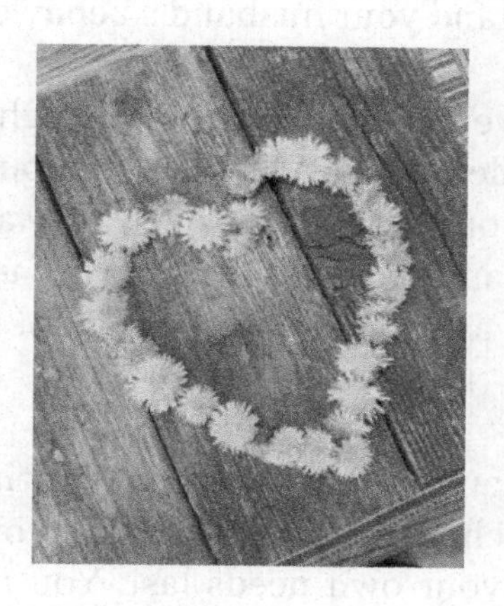

Chapter 8

How to Avoid Caregiver Burnout

It is so important as a caregiver not to become so enmeshed in the role that you lose yourself. It's not good for either you or your loved one.

— Dana Reeve

Providing care and supervision to a person who has dementia can create feelings of stress, burden, guilt, loss, anxiety, and fatigue. Many people worry and wonder if they are doing the right thing, and it is often done in isolation.

Wife caregivers are certainly in the group of isolated or alone caregivers. You may be feeling quite alone in your experience, and it may be difficult for you to ask for or seek help. One of the most important things you can do for yourself is to learn about dementia and caregiving. Education is vital, and, as my grandmother taught me at a young age, knowledge is power. Read everything you can get your hands on in order to be better prepared for what may come your way.

It will help you understand your feelings and frustrations, and it will also help you understand your husband's behaviour.

Sometimes, however, education is not enough. Although you may feel you have a handle on what is going on, you may not be able to *handle* what is going on. Not on your own, anyway. That is where it is important to ask for and receive help. Many of us were never told or taught it is okay to ask for and receive help, so I am giving you permission now.

Self-care of the caregiver involves recognizing when things are getting to be too much. You may feel stressed or overwhelmed, and you may be putting your own needs last. You may be putting your husband's needs first. That is what caregivers tend to do. Think back to when the children were young. A "good mother" always put the needs of her children and family first. I can see how this could carry over into your caregiving role as a wife of a husband who has dementia. That is where we can get into trouble. The stress builds, and we put ourselves at risk of getting sick, both physically and emotionally.

There are ten symptoms of caregiver stress I would like to share here. Consider and reflect on any of the symptoms you are experiencing. This list is adapted from the Alzheimer's Association and Linda Alden (2003):

10 Symptoms of Caregiver Stress or Burnout

1. **Denial** about the disease and its effects on the person who has been diagnosed. "I know he is going to get better."

2. **Anger** at the person with dementia, anger that no cure exists, or anger that people don't understand what's happening. "If he asks me one more time, I'll scream!"

3. **Social withdrawal and isolation**, from friends and activities that once brought pleasure. Lack of interest in personal activities. "I don't care about getting together with the neighbours anymore."

4. **Anxiety** about the future. "What happens when he needs more care than I can provide?"

5. **Depression** or unhappiness that begins to break your spirit and affects your ability to cope. Crying spells. "I don't care anymore."

6. **Sleeplessness and/or Exhaustion** caused by a never-ending list of concerns or feeling under pressure. Completing necessary daily tasks becomes nearly impossible. "What if he wanders out of the house or falls and hurts himself?" or "I'm too tired for this."

7. **Irritability** that leads to moodiness and triggers negative responses and actions. "Leave me alone!"

8. **Lack of concentration** that makes it difficult to perform familiar tasks. "I was so busy; I forgot we had an appointment."

9. **Health problems** that begin to take a mental and physical toll. Headaches, high blood pressure, asthma, nervous stomach, or bowel problems. "I can't remember the last time I felt good."

10. **Withholding affection**, food, bathing, dressing changes for wounds, or medications from the care receiver. Refusing to pay for goods or services under the rationale the expenditures are wasteful on one soon to pass away.

Once we become aware of the symptoms of caregiver stress, we need to pay attention to how we are managing it. Some of us are very good at coping, while others can feel quite immobilized and burdened. Alternatively, you may find yourself engaging in unhealthy ways of coping such as drinking too much alcohol or emotional overeating. In serious cases, depression or anxiety can become quite debilitating. Please consider the following tips for managing stress.

Tips for Managing Stress

- **Know what resources are available** – Home Care, Adult Day Programs (a form of day care for older adults), Paid Caregivers, Meal Delivery Programs, Long-Term Care Homes (see more info in Chapter 7)
- **Ask for help** – Family, friends, Alzheimer's Society, Support Groups, Private Therapists, Dementia Consultants (more detail on this in Chapters 6 & 7)
- **Use relaxation techniques** – Visualization, Meditation, Breathing Exercises, Yoga, Tai Chi
- **Get moving** – Physical activity, walking, gardening, dancing
- **Make time for yourself** – Outings with family and friends, shopping, things you enjoy doing, journaling, laughing, participating in spiritual or religious practices, treating yourself (more on Mini-Vacations to follow)
- **Become an educated caregiver** – Alzheimer's Society and Alzheimer's Association have workshops and helpline (see Chapter 7)
- **Take care of yourself** – Visit the doctor as needed, watch your diet, exercise as able, get plenty of rest and fluids, stay connected with family and friends, keep interested in and learning about the world around you

When help *is* offered, it is important to learn how to *accept* it. Even though it may be difficult to accept the help, saying, "Thank you very much" and allowing the person to assist can be very rewarding. It can help take some of the load off.

The tips are offered as a guide, as you may not need them right now. Understanding what can help minimize and manage caregiver stress can help you a lot as time goes on. There may be other ideas you can think of to add to this list.

Mini-Vacations

Making time for yourself was one of the areas I discussed with the caregiving wives, and they came up with a list of "mini-vacations" they could take. "Mini-Vacations" are physical and/or mental breaks from the responsibilities of caregiving and are an important aspect of self-care. The activities could be as short as a couple of minutes and as long as a couple of weeks. Hopefully these ideas will get you thinking of mini-vacations you can plan for yourself. Here are some ideas from wives who are or have been in your shoes, and they described these times as "Stolen Moments," "Me Time," or "Time to Myself":

- **Reading** – "I'm not here, I am in the story." "I can lose myself in the book." "Takes my mind off of everything." "Helps me relax and fall asleep."
- **Writing** (creative)
- **Journaling** – "I can get out my frustrations." "I don't have to burden anyone."
- **Crossword puzzles**
- **Jigsaw puzzles**
- **Video games** – games on my smartphone, computer, or tablet
- **Crafts** (knitting, crocheting, quilting) – "I like making things and giving them to other people."
- **Work** – "It frees my brain. It's something that is mine. For me, it is a stress-buster. It is good stress."
- **Pajama day** – "A day where I don't have to get dressed or go anywhere."
- **TV** – Sitcoms, soap operas, Cooking Channel, photos, and relaxing music
- **Grocery shopping** – "I enjoy talking to people." "I enjoy browsing."
- **Shopping at the mall or thrift shops** – "I enjoy browsing, not feeling rushed." "It's a peaceful time."
- **Prayer/Meditation**
- **Spiritual or Religious Practices**

No matter what you choose to do, please enjoy it, and remember you have every right to indulge every now and then — even if it is just an ice cream cone from the local fast food outlet! Make time for going out with friends. Spend time with family members whom you like to be with. Treat yourself and take care of yourself.

To end this chapter, I will leave you with "The Caregiver's Bill of Rights" by Jo Horne, author of *Caregiving: Helping an Aging Loved One*, AARP Books (1985).

A Caregiver's Bill of Rights

I have the right:

...to take care of myself. This is not an act of selfishness. It will give me the capability of taking better care of my loved one.

...to seek help from others, even though my loved ones may object. I recognize the limits of my own endurance and strength.

...to maintain facets of my own life that do not include the person I care for, just as I would if he or she were healthy. I know I do everything I reasonably can for this person, and I have the right to do some things just for myself.

...to get angry, be depressed, and express other difficult feelings occasionally.

...to reject any attempts by my loved one (either conscious or unconscious) to manipulate me through guilt and/or depression.

...to receive consideration, affection, forgiveness, and acceptance for what I do, from my loved ones, for as long as I offer these qualities in return.

...to take pride in what I am accomplishing and to applaud the courage it has sometimes taken to meet the needs of my loved one.

...to protect my individuality and my right to make a life for myself that will sustain me in the time when my loved one no longer needs my full-time help.

...to expect and demand that, as new strides are made in finding resources to aid physically and mentally impaired persons in our country, similar strides will be made towards aiding and supporting caregivers.

Exercise:

I can tell I am (or I am not) experiencing caregiver stress because:

____

____

____

I take care of myself by (or I will start to take better care of myself by):

____

____

____

My ideal mini-vacations would be or are:

____

____

____

References:

Alden, Linda (2003). Recognizing and Coping with Caregiver Burnout. *Inside Case Management*. 10.6, p.12.

Alzheimer's Association. (2014). Caregiver Stress. Retrieved from *http://www.alz.org/care/alzheimers-dementia-caregiver-stress-burnout.asp*

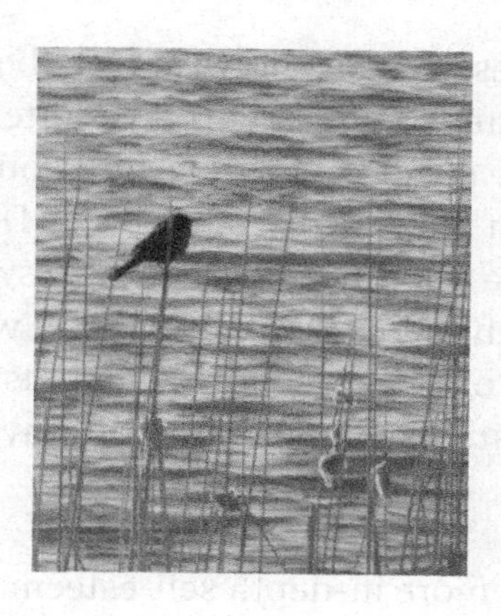

Chapter 9

Improving Self-Esteem

When you're a caregiver, you need to realize that you've got to take care of yourself, because not only are you going to have to rise to the occasion and help someone else, but you have to model for the next generation.

— Naomi Judd

A number of years ago, I developed and facilitated some groups for women on "Self-Esteem" and "Assertiveness." These two topics were very important then, and they continue to be now. Women of every age struggle with issues of self-esteem and assertiveness, and I think it becomes even more important as we age. I would like to talk a little about both of these issues, as it may help you understand yourself and why it is that sometimes you feel unworthy or stressed out.

How We Feel About Ourselves

Self-esteem can be described as how we feel about ourselves. In my work with women and self-esteem, I've often had women ask themselves questions such as: Do you like yourself? Do you treat yourself well? Do you feel worthy of respect? Do you treat yourself kindly as you would a good friend? If they answered "Yes" to these questions or at least answered "Usually," then I would guess they had a good or high level of self-esteem. If they answered "No" or "Not Often" to these questions, then they may have poor or low self-esteem.

If you want to do a more in-depth self-esteem assessment, I would recommend the online version of the "Sorenson Self-Esteem Test." It can be found by putting the title in the Internet search bar. If you score low on this test, you may find low self-esteem is at the root of many of your difficulties. Self-esteem can be improved with education about self-esteem, positive self-talk, and, if needed, psychotherapy or counselling.

As young girls, we receive messages from our parents, our teachers and our peers, as well as society, regarding how we should view ourselves. If we were raised in a family that constantly criticized us or berated us, then it would be difficult to give ourselves permission to like ourselves. The negative criticisms sometimes become our negative self-talk, which may sound something like, "I am never going to amount to anything," or "Nobody likes me." The more negative messages we hear about ourselves, the harder it is to be kind and loving towards ourselves.

On the other hand, if we had very positive feedback from our parents and teachers, and we felt good about our accomplishments and ourselves, we most likely grew up with a positive self-image. This may have resulted in feelings of confidence and self-love, and it was easier to be kind to others and ourselves as a result.

Some women were raised to be "people pleasers." Depending on the culture and family you were raised in, you may have been taught you should never make others unhappy. You may have been told to "Always be mindful of others' feelings." This may have resulted in ignoring your own feelings and needs, which, in turn, may have made you feel resentful.

Passive, Aggressive, and Assertive Behaviour

Assertiveness is the ability to speak up for yourself, while being mindful of others' feelings and opinions. The ability to be respectful of your own needs as well as others' results in assertive behaviours.

There is a spectrum of character traits and behaviours related to this. On one end of the spectrum is Passivity. This is when a person is completely ignorant of his or her own feelings and often is "walked all over." She chooses to do nothing, rather than speak up for herself. The passive person may have low self-esteem or was taught to be a people pleaser and to "not rock the boat."

At the other far end of the spectrum is Aggressiveness. Aggressive behaviour is demonstrated when a person has no respect or consideration for the feelings or needs of others. It may result in abusive or mean behaviour. Shouting, ignoring, and being physically harmful may result. Think of it like bullying behaviour.

There is also Passive-Aggressive behaviour, which can occur when a passive-minded person wants to get her needs met without being overtly or obviously upfront about it. For example, if a woman wanted to go to the store, but her husband did not want her to, she may say something like, "Well, if I don't go to the store, then you won't get your favourite dinner tonight." She is not coming out and saying how she feels, which is most likely controlled; instead, she is using her words as a weapon to hurt her husband's feelings.

Improving How We Feel About Ourselves

In order to overcome some of the problems that poor self-esteem, passivity, and aggressiveness can cause, it is worth keeping some of these thoughts in mind:

- It is healthy, emotionally and mentally, to let the person know how you are feeling, rather than blaming someone else for your problems. A way to communicate your needs goes like this: "I feel ________ when you ____________, and I'd like __________________." Stating how you feel, identifying the behaviour, and then asking for what you want is a simple way to help start the conversation to get situations to change. An example would be, "I feel upset when you don't call me for days, and I'd like you to call me at least every second day, if possible."

- If someone is asking for something from you that you don't want to do, let him/her know politely you can't do it. Tell him/her you are overwhelmed with other things, or things are really busy for you now. Let him/her know how much you would like to be able to help, but the timing is not good. Try to help problem solve and offer suggestions on how she/he could get their needs met by someone else. At the very least, compromise and meet halfway. An example of what you might say would go like this: "I'd really like to help you right now, but I am quite busy with doctors' appointments. Maybe you could ask your friend Joan to help you with that."

- Read books on women and self-esteem. Read about assertiveness. There is a lot of great information out there, in books and on the Internet. Talk to your girlfriends about it. You can learn a lot about the subject and gain a lot of insight.

- To improve your self-esteem, sometimes it helps to write down a list of all the things you are good at and what others have complimented you on. This list of "affirmations" will help you focus on what is positive. You can post these messages on your bathroom mirror or put them in a journal you read daily. I believe what we focus on expands, so if you are constantly berating yourself or thinking negatively about yourself, these thoughts will influence your feelings and behaviours. Therefore, if you have a list of positive things about yourself you repeat once or twice daily, it will help you have happier thoughts, and your behaviour will change.

- A psychotherapist or counsellor can help you work on these issues if you feel you need some professional help in this area.

Becoming aware of our own thoughts, feelings, and behaviours can result in big changes regarding how we operate in this world. Self-reflection, self-compassion, and trying new ways of responding can make a huge difference. Working on improving your self-esteem and learning how to be assertive will most likely result in a reduction in stress, improved confidence, and more peace and contentment in your life.

Exercise:

When it comes to my own self-esteem, I feel:

____

____

____

I would consider (or not consider) myself an assertive person because:

____

____

____

I can try the following to improve my self-esteem and/or assertiveness:

____

____

____

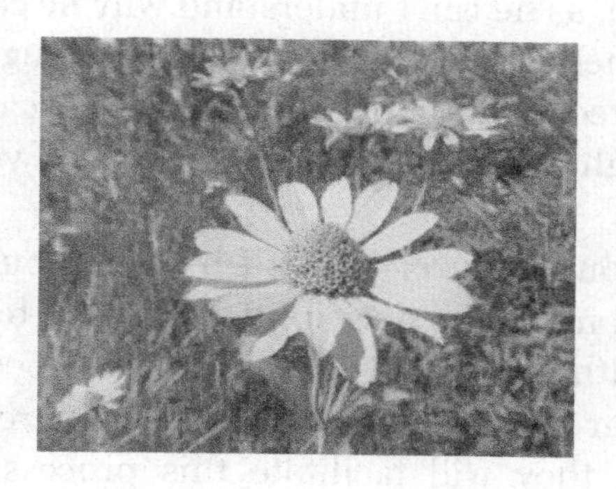

Chapter 10

Long-Term Care Placement

Some days there won't be a song in your heart.
Sing anyway.

— Emory Austin

At some point in your caregiving journey, you may come to the realization that the responsibilities and demands of being a live-in caregiver to your husband are too much for you. You may experience increased stress and worry about how you will keep him safe. Maybe he tries to leave the house without you, and he is at risk of getting lost. Perhaps you have had to call the police a few times already. (More on managing difficult behaviours in Chapter 14). You are getting pressure from your children or friends to have your husband placed into a facility where they can provide a secured environment, with skilled professionals.

Although you feel guilty for having those thoughts, you realize the scale is tipping in favour of having him move to a Home. You are not getting enough sleep. You are exhausted. Maybe you feel like you don't care as much anymore. You are feeling burnt out. You know he would refuse to go, as he can't understand why he can't stay at home anymore. It is something you have to do, even though you don't want to. You have enlisted all the supports at home you can find. However, it still is not enough. Financially, you may worry if you can afford it.

For some of you, the decision will be taken out of your hands. Someone else will make the decision for you. We touched on this in Chapter 4. If health care professionals or other people in authority decide it is in your and your husband's best interests to move into Long-Term Care, they will facilitate this process. If you go into hospital, or if your health is failing, you may not be able to care for him anymore. If his health condition starts to deteriorate, or his dementia is severe, his care may be too complex to manage at home.

Making the Decision

For most situations, one of the first things you need to do is take your husband to the doctor to discuss this option. Hopefully the doctor will be supportive and will help guide you as to how to proceed. He or she may order some blood tests and a chest X-ray to rule out any other medical problems that may be going on.

If the decision is to proceed with Long-Term Care placement, the second thing you will want to do is get in touch with the professionals who will help you make an application. In Manitoba, that is through the Home Care program. Ask about costs. If needed, you may have to apply for an "Involuntary Separation" through Human Resources and Skill Development Canada. This will help adjust the per diem rates (daily costs) for Long-Term Care placement.

Exploring All the Options

If you have disposable income, you will be afforded more options for care. You may want to consider hiring caregivers to look after your husband. There may be privately run Homes you may want to consider. A Geriatric Care Manager may also be able to help you sort out what is needed and what your options are. Still, in the end, you may feel Long-Term Care placement is the best option.

There are other options that may need to be explored, such as Supportive Housing. Long-Term Care Homes provide 24-hour care and supervision, including nursing care. Supportive Housing environments provide 24-hour care but not skilled nursing care. When dementia has progressed to a point where behaviours are quite difficult to manage and require a special approach, a Supportive Housing facility may not be an appropriate housing option.

Generally, a person who has a Mini-Mental State Exam (MMSE) score of 15 or lower would not be appropriate for Supportive Housing. Most people with moderate to advanced or late stages of dementia need to move to a Long-Term Care Home. It is better to move him just once, as it is likely his dementia symptoms will worsen with a move.

Tour Some Homes

Depending on the how the Long-Term Care admissions process works in your health region, you may or may not have a choice of Long-Term Care Home. Manitoba has moved from having three options noted on an application to having only one. This may change in the future. In some health regions, people don't have a choice; rather, they go to the first available spot. Fortunately, there may be an opportunity to transfer to another Home (although the wait may be a year or two, or longer) based on how your Long-Term Care program works.

If you are in an area that allows the opportunity to choose, I would suggest you tour some Homes of your choosing. You may want to ask family or friends for suggestions or the professionals who are helping you with the application process.

Sometimes it helps to pick a Home close to where you live so you don't have to drive so far to see your husband. Pick at least three to tour. You don't have to bring your husband, as this may only upset him. Call the facility, and ask to set up a tour. Sometimes the Social Worker does tours. Write notes about things you liked and did not like about the facility. Ask if they can give you an estimate of how long the wait list is. In the end, you will have some places to choose from.

For more information on how to choose a Home, do an Internet search on "choosing a nursing home" or "selecting a personal care home."

Making the Move

You will most likely be met with resistance from your husband. This is where it is important to rely on your family and friends to help support you through this difficult time. Support Groups could also offer you some great perspectives, as the members of this group can certainly help you know you are not alone in your experience.

You will not be given much notice on a move-in date, so you will have to be ready to act quickly. It is not uncommon to be given a move-in date a day or two later. If the move-in date is too soon, you may be able to delay the actual physical move by agreeing to make payments to secure the spot. This gives you a few more days to make the adjustment.

When the time comes for him to move, you will once again want to enlist help from close family or friends. Pack him up, and bring his medications with him. You will not have to move everything in right away.

Adjusting to the Move

Sometimes the Home may recommend you stay away from the facility for a week or two so your husband is not constantly reminded of his feelings of wanting to go home. The facility will guide you as to the best way to handle the adjustment period. It typically takes between six and eight weeks for someone to adjust to a move, and it takes that long for facility staff to get to know their new residents. He may experience a setback and not be his usual self, but, after an adjustment period, he should return to his normal self. Emotional and behavioural issues may come up, which are expected to sort themselves out with time.

You will most likely go through your own range of feelings, and you, too, will have to adjust to this new arrangement. Your role as caregiver does not stop when your husband moves to a Home. You will continue to provide care, in a different way. You will be considered a valuable part of the team, and you will be invited to meetings. Sometimes you (or another family member) may be called to spend time with your husband when he is feeling unsettled.

He may not remember you have visited him three times this week already, and he may feel very alone. He may not recognize anyone, and he may feel better just hearing your voice on the phone. You will want to attend any special entertainment functions they have so he does not have to attend alone. You will want to report to the nurse anything unusual or alarming that may need to be assessed.

Placing a loved one in a Home is a last resort, and it is a very difficult thing to do. Your role as a caregiver will change, but it will not end at this point. Over the next few months or years, you will be there for him as his condition changes. You may continue to experience ambiguous loss and anticipatory grief (see Chapter 11). You will be comforted knowing you did everything you can for him.

Exercise:

The way I feel about Long-Term Care is:

___

___

___

The way my husband feels about Long-Term Care is:

___

___

___

The cons of caring for my husband at home are:

___

___

___

The pros of my husband moving into Long-Term Care is:

___

___

___

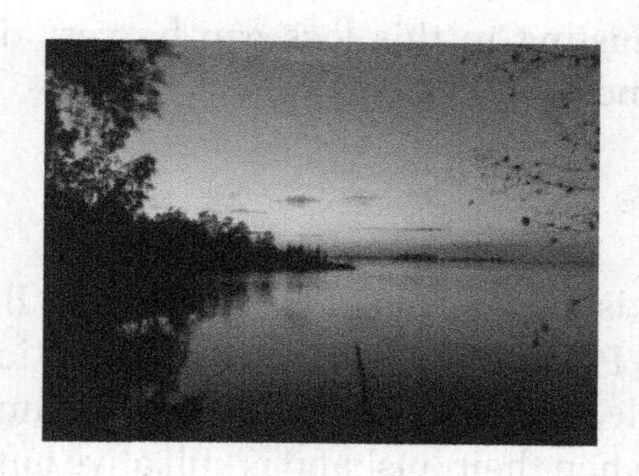

Chapter 11

Loss, Grief, and Bereavement

When someone you love becomes a memory,
the memory becomes a treasure.

— Unknown

When I work with wife caregivers, a concept around grief and loss often appears that I think is quite worthy of discussing here with you. Dementia can rob people of their personality and who they were. It can result in feelings of loss for the people who care about them and love them. The feelings of loss are not always that clear, however, because the loss seems a bit confusing. Your loved one is still physically there, but he is not really the person he used to be.

There are two main types of grief: Living grief and grief after a physical loss. Living grief includes ambiguous loss and anticipatory grief. It has been described as watching a loved one die a little each day, inch by inch.

Death of a loved one is the most stressful life event anyone can endure. Losing a spouse changes your entire life. Widows and widowers have been known to say it is like losing "half" of themselves.

Grief experienced after a loved one dies is called bereavement. Enduring and adjusting to this loss can be very difficult, and, for some, it can become complicated.

Ambiguous Loss

"Ambiguous loss" is a term coined by Dr. Pauline Boss in the 1970s. Some of the wives I work with describe their situation as such: "I feel married, but single," and "I am a widow with a husband." How do these wives cope when their husband is still alive but is "lost" to them as a husband? He is no longer the person he was. How does one cope when a partner is physically present but psychologically absent?

The issue of loss is one most of the women in my program don't feel comfortable talking about. One woman said it was too painful. I got the message early on from the women they were all in different stages of grief.

I know from personal experience how ambiguous loss can feel when a loved one has dementia. The feelings of grief and loss can be strong, even when the person is still alive. It can influence how you interact with the person. You may find yourself crying in his or her presence, and you can't hold back. Even though you try to keep the relationship the same, there is an underlying sadness and fear of the inevitable. You may start to lose hope the person will ever be the same or will ever be able to respond to you like before. You feel your relationship changing, and you start to accept you have lost that person. I look at it as nature's way of helping us say our goodbyes and to let go.

Ambiguous loss needs to be talked about in order for you to understand how your feelings and attitudes are changing towards your husband. The roles will change as his condition changes. Your body and mind are preparing for the reality of the inevitable. The unfortunate reality is you are losing the person who once was. You are losing sight of the future you had planned together.

Anticipatory Grief

You may start anticipating the person's death, a concept known as "Anticipatory Grief." The impending loss may cause you to experience a grief reaction. Elizabeth Kubler-Ross' (1969) five stages of grief include denial and isolation, anger, bargaining, depression, and acceptance. You may start experiencing some of these stages plus additional feelings of dread, anxiety, helplessness, and hopelessness. You may feel guilty and overwhelmed.

Your dreams and hopes of your future with him may start fading away. Even though your husband is still here in body and mind, he is different, and you have to learn how to accept and let go. Hopefully you will have the time to process these feelings, as it is often a slow process. Dementia symptoms may rob your husband of his personality. He may now be but a mere semblance of the person you married.

Give yourself permission to grieve, and be kind to him and yourself as this process unfolds. Even though you may be angry, try not to take your anger out on him. Channel that anger into productive energy like physical activity, or write about your feelings. Talk to a trusted professional or friend. Do not let the anger take over your life. Loss can be a devastating and immobilizing feeling. Give yourself time to process.

Focus on making the most of the time you have left. Check out Dr. Marie Marley's articles found on the internet. She has many helpful tips on how she coped with anticipatory grief in her HuffPost.com article called, "When the End Is Near, What Really Matters?"

End-of-Life Issues

In late-stage dementia, you will most likely have to make decisions about treatment, and you may even have to speak to professionals from Palliative Care or Hospice Care. Your husband may end up going to the hospital to treat life-threatening conditions. You will benefit immensely from relying on the support of other family members during these difficult times.

You may be experiencing ambiguous loss and anticipatory grief while your husband is alive, so, when the time comes that he actually passes away, you may react in a number of ways. Your past relationship with him and dementia severity will affect how you grieve. You may be in shock, and you may not believe it has happened. You may feel guilty you did not do enough for him. You may feel relief, for both him and yourself. You may feel better now that your husband is no longer trapped in a "shell." You may feel guilty for feeling relief, but that is completely normal.

Bereavement

Shortly after your husband passes away, and the reality of your loss has sunk in, you will go through a period of bereavement. The bereaved are those who are left behind after someone has died. You will experience a time of mourning. Some wives will lament, which is when the person who is experiencing the loss may be passionate and very emotional in how she expresses her grief. This is a sad time, and you may feel alone and abandoned.

There is no one "normal" way to experience bereavement. The length of time you grieve and how you express yourself will most likely be influenced by your personality, beliefs, state of mind, and culture. The feelings of grief and loss will lessen with time. You will always miss the person and never forget him, but hopefully you will be able to think of him without crying. Some say you will never "get over" the loss, but the symptoms of grief will recede in time.

Complicated Grief

Some people experience what is called "complicated grief." A loss can trigger sadness, stress, and feelings of abandonment. Sometimes these feelings become quite overwhelming and can continue for quite some time. Grief becomes complicated when it starts to interfere with your daily functioning. The grief may overwhelm you, and life may become too much to handle. You may have trouble finding joy in life. The grieving period may go on for far too long. Although time is passing, you may not feel any less sad. You may feel depressed. You may be having thoughts of death and have a passive wish to die.

If you feel you are not coping well and can't go it alone, consider getting some professional help from a bereavement counsellor. Remember: It is okay to ask for support from your family and friends. Consider joining a support group for people who have lost a spouse. Your doctor or health care professional can help connect you with resources and support.

Your Life Without Him

Some people think they see or hear their deceased loved ones after they have died. This is normal. You may find comfort in keeping some of his personal items, such as a belt, watch, or wallet. You may find yourself crying easily. Anniversaries, birthdays, or other special events could be difficult without him. Ask for support from your family and loved ones.

You want to pay particular attention to making sure you are eating properly and getting enough physical exercise. Ensure you are getting enough sleep. See your doctor as the need arises. Give yourself time to grieve. Hold off on making any major decisions, such as moving, in the first few months. It may take up to a year or more for you to feel better.

To help yourself adjust, you may want to talk with others about your husband and reminisce about your life together. Consider making a photo album of your husband, and share it with family and friends. Get out and get involved in social activities. Consider making new friends or taking up new interests.

It is natural to grieve, and, eventually, a new life will present itself to you. You may then choose to help others deal with this kind of experience, or you may find a completely new life of experiences and opportunities you never expected. Although your caregiving journey will end, a new chapter will begin. You will emerge stronger, wiser, and more capable than ever before.

Exercise:

What can I do to help me prepare for when loss hits me?

____

____

____

What can I do to help myself through the normal grieving process?

____

____

____

References:

Boss, Pauline (2000). *Ambiguous Loss: Learning to Live with Unresolved Grief*. Harvard University Press.

Kubler-Ross, Elizabeth (1969). *On Death and Dying: What the Dying Have to Teach Doctors, Nurses, Clergy, and Their Own Families*. Macmillan Publishing Company.

PART THREE

Practical Tips

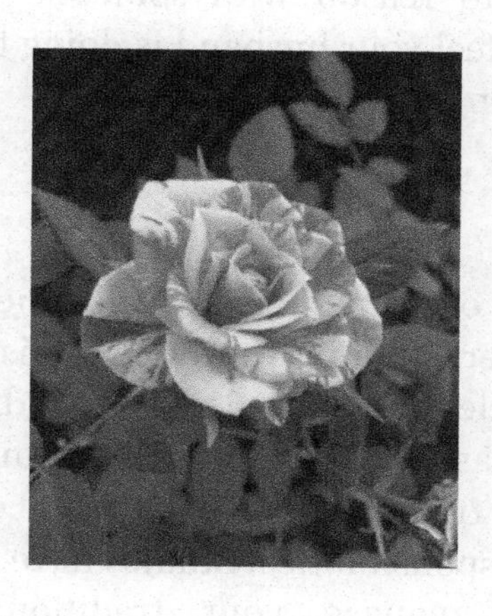

Chapter 12

A New Way of Communicating

Since we cannot change reality,
let us change the eyes which see reality.

— Nikos Kazantzakis

I would hazard to guess you are committed to looking after your husband; otherwise, you would not be reading this book. Your marital vows have most likely played a big role in terms of knowing what your responsibility is, and, as I have heard other wives say, "It's the right thing to do." Some wives have even said, "He would do the same for me if the situation were reversed." This job is tough at times and has been described as a "Lifestyle." I commend you for all you do, and I respect your decision to provide care for your husband as you walk along this journey together.

A common challenge you may experience is communicating with your husband. Dementia affects how a person thinks, acts, and responds, so, at times, it can cause conflict and arguments. There is no point in trying to reason with someone who has dementia. Sometimes you may feel your husband is doing things "on purpose," and this becomes even more frustrating.

Changing Roles

Once the diagnosis of dementia is given and a certain level of acceptance and understanding on your part is achieved, you may want to consider relearning how to talk and interact with your husband. Your role as wife and his as husband are changing and evolving, and, while traditional roles were once held, you begin to take on additional responsibilities. Studies have shown you will most likely continue to manage your traditional roles (such as housekeeping, cooking, cleaning, etc.), but you will most likely also take on the roles that were once held by your husband (such as yard work, taking out the garbage, etc.).

At some point, you may feel your husband is more of a dependent rather than a partner or lover. You may find yourself slipping into a "motherly" role, treating your husband somewhat as a mother treats her child.

Fluctuations Are Normal

Your husband's ability to think and reason rationally will fluctuate. There will be good days and not-so-good days, lucid moments, and confused and disoriented moments. It may be difficult for other people to understand or see what the problems are, because your husband still has the social graces he learned in his earlier, formative years. This is particularly true in cases of Vascular Dementia.

Externalizing Dementia

For some, it helps to "externalize" dementia. A way to do this is to imagine dementia is something that is *affecting* your husband and imagine "removing" it from him. You can do this by imagining him sitting in a chair, cupping your hands around an imaginary entity that is around or in him, and placing it in the air away from him. You can give dementia a name or a metaphor if it helps. A metaphor is a symbol or a representation of something that is more abstract.

Try to imagine your husband is sitting in a chair. Imagine a relationship triangle — you, your husband, and the dementia. The dementia is a *part* of him; it's *affecting* him; it is not *who he is*. In order to work with dementia, you may have to learn how to outsmart it. Externalizing helps depersonalize the upsetting things that happen, knowing it is dementia that is influencing your husband. It is not him, *per se*.

Therapeutic Reasoning®

Under normal circumstances, we would never want to lie to anyone. However, when we are interacting with someone who has dementia, it is by no means "normal circumstances." Dementia is a disease that requires special handling. Sometimes special handling includes the occasional "white lie."

One way to outsmart dementia is by using Therapeutic Reasoning®, a term coined by Dementia Consultant Karen Tyrell. She wrote a book called *Cracking the Dementia Code* (2013), and, in Chapter 8, she states, "Therapeutic Reasoning® is a communication approach used by the caregivers in which they get into the reality of the person with Alzheimer's disease and/or other related dementias in order to 'have a positive benefit for all concerned.'" In other words, it is a type of lying. Therapeutic storytelling has been affectionately referred to as fiblets. Once someone jokingly referred to this type of lying as "morally adjusted truth." It is generally hard (and feels morally wrong) to lie to people, especially loved ones, but if you consider you are lying to the dementia, this may make it easier. It will take practice.

When you lie to someone who has dementia, imagine you are lying *to the dementia*. It is a form of a "white lie," in that it is harmless and trivial. It is meant to avoid hurting someone's feelings or making matters worse. Dementia is not reasonable, and it likes to argue and fight. A way to deal with this sometimes is to "agree" with dementia. As long as it isn't hurting anyone or putting anyone at risk, fiblets can be very helpful (and therapeutic).

Although you may not feel good about lying, if you imagine you are lying *to the dementia* in order to keep the peace, then it may be easier to do. Try refraining from telling your husband he *has to do something*, especially if in the past that has made him react in a negative way. Instead, *suggest* he *may* want to do something (like take a shower) before you. Or, when your husband (actually the dementia) accuses you of taking too long to get the mail (when you were, in fact, talking to the neighbour about how stressed out you are), tell him you are sorry, but you ran into your neighbour who was very upset about her mother's recent hospitalization (Therapeutic Reasoning®). Try out different ways to see what works in your situation. You know your husband best.

Seeking Peace

The end goal is to keep peace in the house and to make your husband feel content. It is not fair to him when dementia and you start arguing. It is not healthy for *your* mental well-being, either. Dementia will never give up.

There is a saying I would like to share with you. It goes like this: "Do you want to be right, or do you want peace?" Since dementia does not know how to reason and take "No" for an answer or take direction very well sometimes, it is a good idea to try therapeutic lying or storytelling to keep the peace.

Try different approaches and techniques. Find out what his triggers are (what upsets him), and avoid them. Learn how to outwit dementia, and see how much more pleasant the situation can be.

Keep a log to see what works and what does not. For more on this concept, search the internet for Dr. Marie Marley's article called, "Do You Want to Be Right or Have Peace?" She gives some good guidelines on how to avoid arguing with someone who has dementia.

Different Ways of Communicating

Try different ways of communicating with your husband, keeping in mind it's the dementia that is influencing his reactions. Experiment with different approaches. Does he like to be *asked* or politely *told* what to do? Example: "Would you like to have your shower before or after me?" or "Could you please put your candy wrappers in the garbage?" Sometimes offering a positive reward or a desired outcome can motivate dementia to get things done. For example, "If you put on a clean pair of pants, we can go to the store and buy your cigarettes." Sometimes your husband's personality will come through, and he will surprise you. Sometimes his personality will be completely different because of the dementia.

Keep your questions, statements, and directions short and sweet. Breaking down complicated steps can also help. For example, "Could you please go to the fridge?" (Wait until he is at the fridge). "Could you please open the freezer?" (Wait until he opens the freezer). "Could you please pull out the chicken and put it on the counter?"

Be mindful of your tone of voice. Although you may be frustrated or upset, it is important to use a loving tone. Dementia often responds well to a loving tone, smiles, and kindness.

You Will Have to Change

You will feel grief and loss of the marital relationship as it was, and you may feel sad about the future and what could have been. You have been given this challenge, and, when you consider you are "dancing with dementia," you may realize you have to change your steps to keep things moving smoothly. One wife said that things improved dramatically *since she changed*. She changed her behaviour and her approach, and it subsequently changed her attitude; it has dramatically decreased her stress level.

Aikido or Validation Technique

Another way to deal with troubling communication patterns is to use a method called "Aikido." The concept of Aikido is taken from a nonaggressive Japanese martial art. It is a form of communication where you pay attention to the *feelings* in a person's message. For example, validating your husband's feelings because you took too long to get the mail can be very comforting. You could say something like, "I sense you are very upset that I took so long," or "Maybe you are upset because you were worried about me?"

Validating or acknowledging feelings can be very comforting to the person who is upset. It helps him/her feel normal and understood. Using an empathetic approach can help deflect any arguments by responding in a caring, nurturing, and nonaggressive way.

Get into His World

Getting into his world is also helpful. Join him and go with it. Sometimes correcting him as to what day it is or who you are does not work and only makes him feel more confused and less sure of himself. Let him feel more in control by getting into his reality and seeing where it takes you. For example, if he sees monkeys outside the window, ask him to talk about the monkeys. Tell him you are surprised there are monkeys out there. Don't deny him his reality, but ask him to share it with you.

Exercise:

The way I view Therapeutic Reasoning® is:

____

____

____

I tried Therapeutic Reasoning®, and:

____

____

____

The benefits of Therapeutic Reasoning® for me are:

____

____

____

Other ways I can change the way I communicate are:

____

____

____

Reference:

Tyrell, Karen (2013). *Cracking the Dementia Code: Creative Solutions to Cope with Changed Behaviours.* Influence Publishing.

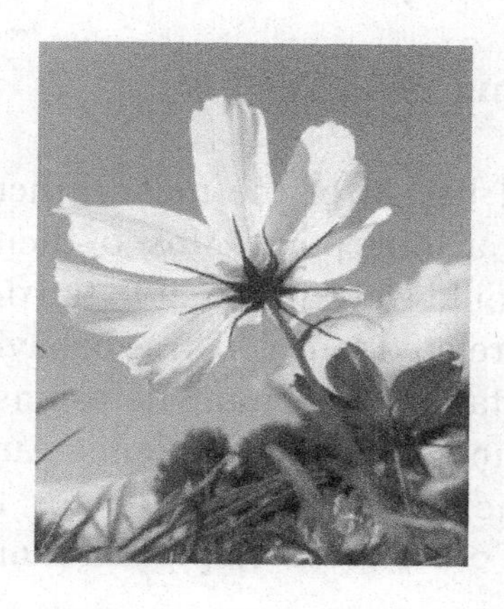

Chapter 13

When to Consult a Physician

The simple act of caring is heroic.

— Edward Albert

When you have a good understanding of what dementia is and you have learned how to deal with the everyday challenges that come up, you may encounter some situations where you are not sure what to do. Your husband will, at some point, lack the insight of knowing when he needs to see a doctor or other health care professional, so you will have to be his eyes and ears.

People living with dementia tend to deny they are having any problems, which will make it tricky for you to assess your husband's health status at times. There are a number of more common symptoms and health concerns to watch for, and these can ultimately cause other problems in behaviour or mood. Keep in mind sometimes the symptoms of dementia can overlap with the symptoms of physical and mental health problems. It is always a good idea to consult a health care professional if you are in doubt.

Behaviour Problems

In Chapter 14, I will list 25 of the most difficult behaviours your husband may exhibit at some point. Most of them, especially if they come on suddenly, would warrant a visit to the doctor to rule out any medical or medicine-related causes. These behaviours and conditions are: Aggression, agitation, delirium, delusions, depressed mood, hallucinating, incontinence, sleep problems. Any of these problems would prompt a phone call or visit to the doctor. In this chapter, I will highlight some of the other common problems and what to look for.

I often refer to the Mayo Clinic website for trusted information (*www.mayoclinic.org*). Here are some of the more common problems seen in older adults you may want to be on the lookout for. This list is not exclusive.

Pain

Your husband may have difficulty expressing his symptoms of pain. If he has a history of chronic pain or a condition such as arthritis, it is quite likely pain will persist, although he may not be able to express himself regarding this issue. You will have to look for signs of pain, like grimacing, groaning, or moaning. He may limit his activities or avoid doing certain movements. Uncontrolled pain, even a headache, for example, can cause a person with dementia to feel agitated or irritable.

Urinary Tract Infections

The urinary tract can become infected and cause discomfort and other problems. There are three main areas that can become infected: kidneys, bladder, and urethra. Each area will have its own set of symptoms. Symptoms such as burning on urination, frequent and painful urination, or back or side pain can indicate a problem. When your husband has problems with holding his urine, and he becomes incontinent, he may have a bladder infection. He may feel burning on urination (urethra infection), or he may have a fever (kidney infection).

If left untreated, a urinary tract infection (UTI) can cause more problems and can ultimately lead to a systemic infection called sepsis. A UTI is easily diagnosed by a simple urine test and is most often easily treated with antibiotics. Occasionally frequent infections require a different course of treatment, and severe infections may require intravenous antibiotics in the hospital. Check out the info on the Mayo Clinic website (*www.mayoclinic.org*) for more details if required.

Reaction to Medication

If your husband has been prescribed a new medication, it can cause side effects that may change his behaviour. He may have an upset stomach, for example, or he may become delirious (altered thinking or attention). A simple eye drop prescription has been known to cause delirium in some people. Stopping it will not cure the dementia but improve the situation to the previous level of impairment prior to when the new medication was started.

Suddenly stopping medications, running out of pills, or forgetting to take them can also cause changes in behaviour. Anti-depressant and anti-anxiety medications can cause untoward side effects if stopped abruptly. It is always wise to consult with a doctor or pharmacist regarding stopping medications. Another common medication many people have a reaction to is antibiotics. Antihistamines can also cause problems. Chapter 14 has more information on what medications to watch for.

Increase in Drowsiness

If your husband has a sudden need to sleep all day, you would be well advised to speak to the doctor about this. This could be a health-related problem (such as blood iron deficiency or hypothyroidism) or a mood-related problem (such as depression). It could also be a reaction to medication.

As I mentioned previously, you may want to be more observant of your husband's behaviour and mood in order to prevent something more serious. Pay particular attention to any sudden changes.

Exercise:

My husband is prone to the following conditions:

____

____

____

When I tell my husband I would like him to go to the doctor, he says:

____

____

____

The way I get him to go to the doctor is:

____

____

____

What I want to ask or tell the doctor is:

____

____

____

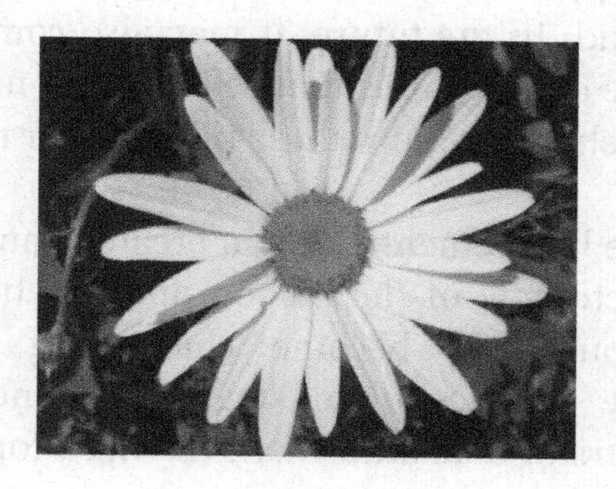

Chapter 14

Coping with Difficult Behaviours

I understand why Alzheimer's caregivers can be so thoroughly disconcerted day after day. We don't know how long. We don't know what is coming next. We feel like we are walking 'up the down staircase' each and every day.

— Bob DeMarco

First, take a deep breath. Then take another one.

If you are reading this chapter, then you may be facing some very difficult times. You may want to refer to this chapter often. Consider this chapter as a reference guide. You need to read only the sections that pertain to you, in your situation. There will be parts you won't need to read, at least not for now. You may need to skim through though, so you know what is contained in this chapter if you should require it.

These tips are also available in a smartphone application (app) called, "Dementia Caregiver Solutions." Dementia Consultant Karen Tyrell worked with me on the app and the information contained in this chapter. The app can be found at the App Store for those who use iPhone and/or iPad. In the future, it may also come in an Android version. Check the online stores that sell apps for mobile devices for availability if you should require these tips on your mobile device.

When someone has dementia, it can create changes in behaviour that are uncharacteristic of the person and can be problematic to manage. Behaviours can become challenging and sometimes dangerous in the middle-to-late stages of dementia. Often the problem behaviours of dementia cause the need for specialized care in a long-term care home.

Long-term care placement is a last-resort option. Most people want to avoid it all together, but sometimes it is necessary. You want your husband home as long as possible, and he most likely prefers to stay in his familiar environment. Whether that decision or desire is motivated by love, guilt, finances, or something else, you have every right to feel what you feel.

While you contemplate or wait for placement, you may have to deal with some challenging behaviours, depending on how long you need to wait. Note difficult behaviours can continue in the long-term care home, and new behaviours can appear along the journey.

Behaviour Management Worksheet

A simple technique used to help with most behaviour problems is developing a "Behaviour Management" worksheet. The heading is the target behaviour, such as, "Refuses to Change Clothes." The worksheet has five columns bearing the following headings:

1. Date
2. Time
3. Triggers — What was happening before?
4. Tried — What did you try?
5. Outcome — Did it work? / What happened?

Here is an example of what your form may look like:

Target Behaviour: ______________________________

Date	Time	Triggers	Tried	Outcomes

This form can be used with any type of challenging behaviour. For example, if you have been having difficulty getting your husband to agree to change his clothes, you may want to read about strategies that may work better for both of you (suggestions can be found in the following section). Your intervention may be to try laying out his clothes in the order they are to be put on. You then note this on your Behaviour Management worksheet and include the date, time, what was happening before the behaviour, what you tried, and what the outcome was. If it worked, you can try it again. If it didn't, you can try a different technique.

Behavioural and Psychological Symptoms

When a person with dementia enters middle stages, sometimes his ability to understand and cope in his environment becomes difficult. The medical terms for the symptoms unique to dementia, are called "Behavioural and Psychological Symptoms of Dementia" (BPSD). They have also been referred to as challenging, difficult, unwanted, disruptive, negative, or problem behaviours.

Health care professionals knowledgeable in the field of dementia may refer to the behaviours as "reactive" or "responsive." There is a greater understanding the person with dementia is responding or reacting to either stimuli in his/her environment or to other people. He or she may be reacting to an unmet need (such as being in pain or being hungry). It is also my understanding there is a reason or trigger for all behaviour, and it doesn't come "out of the blue."

The best approach to managing BPSD is by educating caregivers and using individualized techniques and approaches. You cannot change the behaviour of your husband, so it would be helpful to learn how to change your own approaches and reactions. Sometimes the environment needs to be changed. Once we understand and apply this concept, the situation has a much better chance of improving. The most important thing to remember is the person is not doing things to you on purpose. Dementia is affecting his behaviour.

Medications and Problem Behaviour

Medications are often prescribed to "treat" problematic behaviours. There is a lot of valid concern over the safety of these medications. Atypical antipsychotics (sedatives or major tranquilizers) and hypnotics (especially sleeping pills or anti-anxiety medications) must be used with caution, and all of the risks and benefits must be considered prior to use. Some of these medications have "Black Box" warnings, so you may want to discuss your concerns with the doctor or a pharmacist. A geriatric specialist (a doctor who specializes in working with older people) would also be a great resource for this area of concern.

"Beers (not the drink) Criteria" sets out recommendations for potentially inappropriate medication use in older adults. As an example, with regard to antipsychotics, "Avoid use for behavioural problems of dementia unless nonpharmacologic options have failed and patient is a threat to self or others."

For more information on Beers Criteria, American Geriatrics: Visit *https://www.americangeriatrics.org* and search "Beers" for the latest information.

25 Difficult Behaviours

In the next section, you will find information on the 25 most difficult dementia-related behaviours, including the definition of the problem and a list of possible solutions. My hope is that it will inspire you to think creatively and generate ideas that are personalized to your situation. Some techniques may work some of the time, and the situation is likely to change over time, so it is always a good idea to be open to new ideas. Patience and creativity can pay off. (These behaviours can affect both men and women, but for purposes of this book, I will refer to men only.)

Tips for these situations follow:

1. Aggression
2. Anxiety/Agitation
3. Bathing
4. Catastrophic Reactions
5. Delirium
6. Delusions
7. Depressed Mood
8. Doesn't Recognize Others
9. Doesn't Recognize Self
10. Dressing
11. Hallucinating
12. Hiding Possessions
13. Inactivity
14. Incontinence
15. Poor Eating Habits
16. Refusing Care
17. Repetition
18. Repetitive Sounds
19. Rummaging/ Hoarding
20. Sexual Expression
21. Sleep Problems
22. Sundowning
23. Unsafe Driving
24. Wandering
25. Wants to "Go home"

Keep in mind these guiding principles with respect to managing difficult behaviours:

- Never argue with someone with dementia. He is not capable of reasoning and logic.

- Use Therapeutic Reasoning® or other techniques for communicating as mentioned in Chapter 12.

- Talk to the doctor if there is a concern.

- Always use a soothing and calm tone of voice.

- Always be on the lookout for what may be causing the behaviour. Every case will be different.

1. Aggression (Verbal and Physical)

Problem: When a person is upset or frustrated, or feels a lack of control in the environment, he may use verbal aggression. He may argue, swear, belittle, yell, or become threatening. It may escalate to physical aggression, and he may punch, hit, slap, kick, or throw things.

Solutions:

- Stay calm, and speak in a quiet, soothing voice.

- Leave the room. Call for help if you feel you are at risk of being harmed.

- Don't argue back. This will only escalate the situation.

- Remove objects that are sharp or dangerous and may potentially be used as a weapon.

- If he has something in his hand you would like him to put down, calmly and politely ask him to give you the item or put it down.

- Give him some personal space. Ask him if he wants to be left alone for a while (cool-down period).

- You may try Therapeutic Reasoning® to help divert a crisis. You can apologize or say you will look into fixing things.

- Let the doctor know if his behaviour is becoming unmanageable and/or dangerous. He may require a physical assessment and a review of his medication.

- Let him vent when you are at a safe distance.

- When there is a break, respond to and validate his feelings, not the behaviour.

- If there is a high risk for violence, keep a jacket by the door with keys, driver's license and money, so you can leave quickly in an emergency.

- In an extreme case, if you are in immediate danger, leave the home and call the police.

- When he is calmed down, ask him to tell you what happened, and try to find a solution and prevent it from happening again.

2. Anxiety/Agitation

Problem: The person appears restless and unsettled. He is not easily consoled. He may feel like fidgeting and moving around, and he can't sit still. He may also feel irritated and easily annoyed. He may say he feels "on edge." He may feel fear, nervousness, or unease. Anxiety is the feeling, while agitation is the behaviour.

Solutions:

- Seek the reason he became agitated, and then offer support accordingly.

- Find out what he is nervous or concerned about by asking him.

- Provide reassurance as much as you can (even if you need to use Therapeutic Reasoning®).

- Show you are concerned about his needs/issues.

- Ask him to talk about how he is feeling.
- Validate his feelings.

- Let the doctor know if the agitation or anxiety is getting worse. The person may require a physical assessment and a medication review.

- Speak in a calm, soothing, pleasant voice.

- Let him know you are there to help him. Ask him, “Is there something I could do to help?”

- Ask if he needs to use the washroom or if he is hungry, tired, or cold. (Think physical concerns.)

- Quiet the immediate area, or take him to a quieter room.

- Suggest he lie down in a quiet room.

- Offer him a shoulder or back rub.

- Play some relaxing music.

- Put on his favourite TV program or video. This offers a diversion from his current state.

- One on one may be more comforting than talking in a group.

- Try reminiscing.

- Encourage a visit with a pet or a child.

- Offer/suggest a walk to get some fresh air.

- Try giving him a 10-minute aromatherapy (fragranced or aromatic) hand massage.

3. Bathing

Problem: The person does not want to have a bath or shower.

Solutions:

- Try to determine the reason he doesn't want to have a bath or shower.

- Ask him his reasons for not wanting to take a bath or shower. Then alter your response/actions.

- Determine how often is necessary. For example, incontinence (bowel or bladder) or poor daily hygiene habits would require more frequent baths/showers.

- Try to keep the bath or shower routine as close to his usual habits as possible (e.g., a shower in the morning or a bath at night).

- Pick a time when he is already doing a related activity, like getting changed or using the toilet.

- Have someone else suggest he have a bath.

- Remind him how good he felt after having his last shower.

- Ask him if he *prefers* a bath or a shower, rather than saying *it is time* for his bath/shower; then proceed to get the towels and soap ready and water running. This approach provides him with a choice.

- If he wants to go out somewhere, let him know you will go right after he bathes and gets ready to go. Sometimes incentives work.

- If he adamantly refuses, leave and come back later. Sometimes a different approach at a different time works.

- Encourage a sponge bath, also known as "top and tail" or "bird bath" on other days.

- Install a handheld shower nozzle, and provide a bath seat or bench for safety. Grab bars are also reassuring.

- If he is afraid of falling, put in a non-slip mat, and help him in and out of the tub.

- Have someone else provide this assistance, such as a paid caregiver or other family member. Find out if the provincial government Home Care program can assess for eligibility.

- Suggest going to get a hair wash at a salon.

- Try creating a coupon that indicates, "Good for one free beauty makeover" and express how lucky he is.

- Check to see if your local Adult Day Program services include bathing.

- If he is capable of showering or bathing on his own, adjust the temperature on the hot water tank to prevent him from scalding himself.

- Offer a distraction in the shower/bath such as a face cloth or hand towel to hold if you are doing most of the assisting.

- If he likes music, have music playing while you are assisting him, and maybe sing along together.

- Explain step by step what you are going to do.

- Explain who you are and what you are going to do if he has difficulty remembering who you are. Extra reassurance may go a long way.

- Be sure the temperature of the room is to his liking.

- If he complains often about how cold it is in the shower, try to warm up the room before you have him undress. Have a warm towel ready to go when the water stops. Warm up a towel in the dryer just before the bath/shower.

- If privacy is an issue, have him cover up with a towel to feel secure. Having an extra wet towel may be a minor inconvenience compared to the other challenges you may experience.

- Show patience and a soft, caring smile throughout the bathing experience.

4. Catastrophic Reactions (Overreacting)

Problem: The emotional reaction is exaggerated and doesn't match the situation. The person is not easily settled. He may throw things, yell, and appear very angry or upset. It is best to consider the reason for this behaviour (trigger) and work on avoiding it.

Solutions:

- Remain calm. Take a deep breath, and remind yourself it is not him but rather the symptoms of dementia.
- Speak in a soothing, quiet manner.
- Keep at arm's length if you feel you are at risk of getting hit or hurt.
- Avoid getting angry at him.
- Try to understand his reasons for this behaviour.
- Validate his feelings and help him feel understood.
- Make sure the area is safe and others are safe.
- Remove sharp or dangerous objects.
- Respect personal space, and keep a safe distance until the episode has passed.
- Do not use touch unless you know for certain touch will calm him.
- Remove the stressor, if possible.
- Help him move to a quieter area, if possible.
- Never argue with someone who has dementia, especially in this state; rather, agree and validate his feelings.

- You may try Therapeutic Reasoning® to help de-escalate a crisis. For example, if he insists your son took the envelope with money from his wallet, simply agree and say you understand how upset he is and you are going to help him to make it right.

- Don't rush him.

- Give him a lot of time to prepare for the next activity.

- Learn what the triggers (causes) are, and try to avoid them.

- Learn from this event so you can prevent it from happening again.

- Share with others who provide him care, so this situation may be avoided.

- To prevent catastrophic reactions, try to stick to a familiar routine, ensure he is well rested, and speak in a way he can understand.

5. Delirium

Problem: A person who has dementia is at a greater risk of developing delirium. Delirium usually begins suddenly, and it can fluctuate in severity. Delirium can last days or months. A person who is delirious will present as very confused, may hallucinate, and become very agitated or irritable. Alertness levels will fluctuate, and he may mix up his days and nights. Common causes of delirium include dehydration, infection, pain, and certain medications. Delirium in older adults is considered a medical emergency as it affects thinking and attention. It can increase the need for care, supervision, or hospitalization. It can increase the risk of disease and/or death.

Solutions:

- A sudden change in a person's behaviour or worsening confusion can be a sign of delirium. It is important to have a doctor assess the person. A review of blood tests, urinalysis, medications, checking for skin infections, pain in the body, etc., would be very important.

- A person who is delirious will have a fluctuation in his ability to concentrate. He will need more assistance during this time.

- He may experience hallucinations or delusions and will require some extra reassurance that he is safe.

- Ensure the delirious person is comfortable, hydrated, and well supervised. Watch for signs of worsening in his condition.

- You may want to enlist the help of others for this time period so you don't experience burnout.

- If new medications are prescribed, for example, for a urinary tract infection, ensure the medications are taken as prescribed, and watch for further signs of side effects.

- Contact the doctor if his condition does not improve or worsens.

- Ensure his needs are responded to as he recovers.

- Be sure to do follow-up tests, as it is common for some infections to return, even after treatment with antibiotics.

6. Delusions (False Beliefs)

Problem: The person has a fixed, false belief that cannot be changed by reasoning or logic. He may think someone is trying to harm him or take his things. Sometimes he thinks people are watching him or replacing his things.

Solutions:

- A sudden onset of delusions or paranoia can be a symptom of a medical problem such as delirium or a reaction to medication. Consider making a doctor's appointment for assessment.

- Try to determine the root cause for the delirium.

- Do not challenge his beliefs. Reasoning does not often work and may cause arguments or conflict. Agree with his feelings and the concept.

- Say things like, "I believe you are convinced this is happening to you, and it must be upsetting. I know I would be upset if that happened to me."

- Reassure him you will help in any way you can, and remind him he is safe.

- Ask him what he thinks you should do to help the situation.

- Try distraction or diversion techniques by changing the subject and having him think about something else. Keep him occupied with other activities.

- Apologize by saying, "I am sorry to see you are upset by this" as a way to help calm the situation.

7. Depressed Mood

Problem: People can become depressed at any stage in life, and this can negatively affect mood, appetite, sleep habits, motivation, and social activity. They can appear sad, crying, unmotivated.

Solutions:

- Ask him why he is looking sad.
- Validate his feelings.
- You may want to suggest an appointment with a counsellor.
- Consider getting him to see a doctor for a medical assessment and to discuss treatment options.
- Go for a walk together, and make sure he gets some sunlight.
- Exercise of any kind can make a difference.
- Encourage him to be sociable, such as by attending family gatherings or social events. Also, be mindful he may like to see only one visitor at a time or feel more comfortable in smaller groups.
- Give him a purpose. Ask him to help out with a responsibility in the house he can safely manage, for example, shredding papers, sweeping floors, dusting railings, or folding towels. To help him feel needed and useful, recognize his efforts, thank him, and show appreciation with a smile of gratitude.
- Ask him to talk about his thoughts and feelings. Let him know it is okay to feel sad and it is okay to cry if he wants to.
- Take him on a shopping trip or for a country drive.

- Play some of his favourite music.
- Offer a shoulder or back rub.
- Try giving him a 10-minute aromatherapy (fragranced or aromatic) hand massage.
- If he is having suicidal thoughts, immediately seek help from a doctor or mental health professional.

8. Doesn't Recognize Others

Problem: Dementia may cause the person to not recognize his own children or spouse. He may mistake you for someone else. This can be very upsetting for a family member or spouse. Although it can be distressing for you, he may still enjoy your company, and that is what matters.

Solutions:

- Gently correcting or reorienting him may help, but it may also make him feel more confused or unsure of himself. Gauge if this is a good way to approach this problem.
- Reassure him you are someone he can trust and you have known him for a long time.
- Put yourself into context. Remind him how you know him, and bring up some memories from long ago. This may help him connect with you.
- Show him some photos of you and him together. Show him old photos of you.
- Let him know you love him and you like having him around.

- If he is asking about or wanting to know the whereabouts of someone who has passed on, such as his mother, just "go with it" to keep the peace. Ask him where this person would normally be on a day like today. If he is certain this person is still around and wants to speak to him/her, say you will look into it. To be more convincing, you might try to "phone" the person and say it looks like he/she is not home right now, but you can try calling later. Then offer a diversion of some other pleasant activity. This Therapeutic Reasoning® is done to help, not to cause harm; it may prevent him from becoming upset.

- He may remember the sound of voices but not appearances. Experiment with him talking on the phone. Try talking to him from another room, as this may help.

9. Doesn't Recognize Self

Problem: Dementia may rob the person of his ability to recognize himself in the mirror. He may recognize only a younger version of himself. This can cause fear and confusion. This is called agnosia.

Solutions:

- Cover up or remove mirrors. (Ideas: curtains, turning sliding doors around, or customized plastic wrapping the area.)

- When the sun starts to set, close drapes and/or blinds to minimize reflections in windows.

- Offer reassurance and respond to the feelings if he is concerned or upset by the "old man" in the mirror/house.

10. Dressing

Problem: He might refuse assistance with changing clothes, getting ready for bed, or putting on clean underwear, believing he can do it himself.

Solutions:

- Ensure privacy at all times. Most people are very shy undressing in front of others.
- Have only one body part exposed at a time.
- Minimize clutter, and remove unused clothes from the closet.
- If he has trouble choosing what to wear, help him by offering some suggestions.
- To minimize confusion, try limiting outfit choices to two.
- Ask him why he does not want to get dressed today.
- Ask him what time he would like to (or plans to) get dressed.
- Let him know you would like him to get dressed after his show, or in 15 minutes, for example.
- In a caring voice, let him know, if he would like, you are happy to assist him with getting dressed.
- Offer to assist him with only one small task in the dressing process (the part he seems to have most difficulty with). If he refuses, do not insist. Avoid a crisis. (If he reacts, go back to the section on Catastrophic Reactions to learn other techniques.) You may want to try again at a different time.

- If he gets agitated while you are helping him, you may need to walk away. Perhaps tell him you have something to attend to and you will be back in a few minutes. Return and see if it is better timing.

- Set out his clothes if he needs help with this task.

- Lay out the clothing in the order they are to be put on, with undergarments on top.

- If he needs cueing assistance, tell him what item to start with, and let him know you will help him along. Hand him one item at a time.

- If buttons are too difficult to manage, try using pullovers or t-shirts. Zip-front cardigans may also be worth a try. Clothing and shoes that fasten with Velcro may help.

- You may want to try saying company is coming, and you noticed he has a bit of a food stain on his shirt (or pants); maybe he would like to get changed.

- Tell him about the special treat (food or objects he enjoys) you will have ready for him after he gets dressed. (Incentives sometimes work.)

- If he is agitated or frustrated with the situation, reassure him in a calm voice he will feel better once he gets ready for the day, or bed, or whatever.

- Distract from the activity of helping him by talking about things that interest him or singing a song. Maybe he will forget you are helping him, and the task will no longer be the focus.

- When he gets undressed for his bath, remove his dirty clothes and put them in the wash or out of sight as soon as possible. Be sure the clean clothes are there for him to see.

- If he has a favourite colour and/or style of clothing, you may want to buy multiples. That way, he will always have a familiar clean item handy.

11. Hallucinating

Problem: Some people see, hear, taste, or feel things that are not real. It could be because of a medical problem or a process in the brain that is affected by dementia. This is called hallucinating. A related condition is a person misinterpreting something that is actually there. This is called an illusion.

Solutions:

- A sudden onset of hallucinations could indicate a medical problem, such as delirium. Consider making an appointment with a doctor or mental health professional.

- Reassure the person he is safe, and let him tell you what he saw or heard.

- Validate his feelings. "I can see you look worried about this. Can you tell me more about what is going on?"

- Show interest in what he sees, and ask questions about it. Ask him questions such as "How many?" or "How often?"

- Remain calm and understanding. Respond to the feelings he may be expressing. Say, "It sounds like you are upset that you saw these people in your living room."

- Reassure him he is safe. Say things like, "You are safe here," "I will look after this," "Would it be okay if I gave you a hug?" or "Can I hold your hand?"

- If it appears to be an illusion (an inaccurate perception or a misinterpretation of information), try removing the object that is causing him to "see" something else, or move it to another room.

- Make sure his glasses are clean. Arrange an eye exam if needed.

- Make sure his hearing aids are working properly.

- Offer to take him out, go for a coffee, or stop at a mall.

12. Hiding Possessions

Problem: When people have memory problems, it is common for them to misplace their possessions. When this happens, they may assume someone has stolen from them. Their fears and suspicion then cause them to want to hide their things in a safe spot. Then, they forget where they put them. What results is a cycle of frustration for the person with dementia and the caregivers.

Solutions:

- Remove valuables and store in a safe-deposit box or other safe place. Let him know you have it and will guard it for him.

- Give him small amounts of cash, so if he loses or misplaces it, it will be only a small amount.

- Remove all of the important papers from his wallet, to ensure valuable or important documents are safe.

- Help him find his lost or stolen items and reassure him everything is okay. Validate his feelings of loss, victimization, and violation.

- Provide him with multiples of the items he often misplaces (glasses, wallet, purse, etc.).

- If losing keys is a problem, make sure you have a spare set. Give him a lanyard (thick string necklace to attach his keys to) or a wearable wrist key coil so he always has his keys with him.

- Try using a "smart key" or "wireless sensor tag" system. These gadgets are paired with a mobile device or a computer, and the location of the tagged item can be determined.

- Check wastebaskets before throwing away any garbage bags.

- Downsize the living area in the house by eliminating access to specific rooms or storage closets.

- Remove clutter and extra storage space to reduce the time it may take to find things.

- Reassure him you will help. Maybe say, "I'm not sure what happened, but I will look for it" or "I am looking into it."

- If he is upset about losing an item and he cannot be consoled, he may experience a catastrophic reaction (see: Catastrophic Reactions). Watch for signs, and help divert a crisis if you can.

13. Inactivity

Problem: There are times when a person with dementia is content to do nothing but sit or sleep. They become listless. He is not necessarily depressed or bored; he just doesn't do anything. He no longer initiates activities. It may be too much for him to organize himself to do things he used to do. He appears apathetic (does not appear interested or enthusiastic).

Solutions:

- Ask him how he is feeling. Is he tired or feeling any pain? Does he have a headache?
- Consider if this change is related to depressed feelings. Seek a doctor for support on this.
- Try to get him engaged in talking about things that normally interest him, such as positive events from the past.
- Try going through family photo albums, or put on family home videos to spark engagement.
- Ask him to come for a walk with you. Tell him you would like some company.
- Tell him you want to go for a drive, and you don't want to go alone. Point out some interesting sights.
- Play some of his favourite music.
- Try giving him a 10-minute aromatherapy hand massage.
- Offer him a snack. Have him assist a little with this activity.

- Give him an activity that is purposeful yet simple, safe, and repetitive. Make it appear as though it is a much-needed task and you would really appreciate his assistance. Ideas: Shredding papers for local animal shelters or even sanding wood blocks for a day care.

- If he becomes upset with your suggestions, back off. Try again at a different time.

- Look into an Adult Day Care Service that specializes in dementia or memory care with a program that will offer him a change of scenery and to socializing with others. Eligibility and costs vary across jurisdictions.

14. Incontinence

Problem: Sometimes it becomes difficult to manage elimination (bladder or bowels) as dementia progresses. There are times when the person is incontinent of urine and refuses to wear protection, or a man may choose to urinate in an inappropriate spot, like a planter. This adds to the person's embarrassment, and he may refuse to be helped. A confused person may have a bowel movement in his undergarments and then try to clean it up himself, causing more mess and humiliation.

Solutions:

- Check with the doctor to make sure there is no urinary tract infection or other medical problem with his prostate. Having a bladder infection can cause incontinence or urgency (the urgent need to get to the toilet).

- When you are home with him, encourage him to use the toilet every two to three hours. This is called a toileting schedule or routine. If he cannot go by himself, offer to assist him.

- Make sure his clothes are easy to remove. Elasticized waistbands make pants easy to manage.

- If he refuses to wear incontinence products, you may try to replace all of his underwear in his drawer with only disposable, absorbent pull-ups. They look like underpants, and he may put them on if there is no other alternative.

- Ensure he is changing his brief when it is soiled. If he refuses help from you, then you may want to consider having someone else do it, such as a private-duty home care worker.

- Consider having a Home Care assessment (some countries, like Canada, have publicly funded programs) to see if he is eligible for services that could assist him throughout the day.

- Remove soiled clothing to help keep the odour under control.
- Check the bedding to ensure it is also kept clean.
- Purchase soaker pads for the bed if there are problems with nighttime incontinence. There are also waterproof mattress pad covers available.

- Put a urinal or commode by the bedside if nighttime proves to be a problem.

15. Poor Eating Habits

Problem: He is not eating as much as he should, or he is not eating the right kinds of foods for good nutrition. Sometimes he forgets to eat. In addition, he is losing weight. Alternatively, he may want to eat all the time.

Solutions:

- Try to determine why his eating habits have changed.
- Does he have pain in his mouth? A toothache or other problem? A visit to the dentist may help.
- If he wears dentures, are they fitting properly?
- Does he have a stomach upset such as an ulcer?
- Ask him questions such as, "Please tell me the reason you don't want to eat today."
- Offer frequent small meals during the day.
- Try keeping a scheduled meal routine if this helps.
- If you are not with him, call him to remind him to eat the meal you prepared for him.
- Ensure there are plenty of healthy foods available, such as fruit and salad.
- Provide or encourage fluids throughout the day to prevent dehydration.
- Offer his favourite foods as often as possible.
- Offer a choice of meals rather than decide for him.
- Eat together, if possible, as meal times are best shared with others.

- Try finger foods, if using utensils is too difficult for him to manage.
- If he has trouble seeing white food on a white plate, try a different coloured plate. (Many people have had success with the colour red.)
- Seek out a dietician or occupational therapist if you are still having trouble getting him to eat. It may be time to change the texture of his meals.
- Consider using a nutritional supplement between meal times (such as Ensure or Boost).
- Try homemade smoothies, using food items he enjoys.
- Help him eat by providing cueing, encouragement, or physical assistance. For example, place food on his fork, place the fork in his dominant hand, and cue him to put the fork up to his mouth.
- Consider having someone else make and encourage his meals.
- Check into home-delivered meal programs (e.g., "Meals on Wheels").
- Hire private-duty home care workers to provide meal assistance.
- If sitting for meals is a problem, provide healthy snacks throughout the day.

16. Refusing Care

Problem: He might refuse assistance with bathing, dressing, grooming, or medications. He often believes he can do it himself or he did it already. The reality is, if he does not have assistance or at least cueing, he is at risk of self-neglect.

Solutions:

- Offer to assist with the task. If he refuses, come back at a different time.

- Offer validation. Try saying, "I know you don't like it when we do this. To be honest, neither do I. How about we do it as fast as we can so we can go on to do something else?"

- With a smile, try gently *telling* him (versus asking him) it is time for his bath/medications/clothing change, and proceed with instructing him as to what you are doing and what you expect from him.

- Give the person a choice as to what to wear or what time he wants to get dressed, for example (see: Dressing).

- Put out the medications and a glass of water, and allow him to take them on his own, if capable. If he does not take them this way, try reminding him what the medication is for and his doctor wants him to take them to keep him healthy and strong.

- Some medications can be crushed or liquefied and put into his food. Ask your pharmacist.

- If he is agitated or frustrated with the situation, reassure him he will feel better once he is dressed, or shaved, or whatever.

- Remind him it will only take a moment and you will leave him alone after.

- If he gets agitated while you are helping him, tell him you have something to attend to and you will be back in a few minutes. Return to see if it is a better time to try again.

- While you help him, distract from the activity by talking about things that interest him, or even try singing a song. Maybe he'll forget you are helping him, and the task will no longer be the focus.

- Break the care activity into small steps with a break in between.

- Consider spreading the tasks out during the day. For example, clipping his fingernails several hours after his bath.

17. Repetition

Problem: The person tends to repeat things, ask the same questions repeatedly, or tends to engage in repetitive behaviours. He cannot remember he asked the question already, and he cannot remember the answer. He may repeat certain behaviours because they are familiar.

Solutions:

- Try to determine the reason for the repetition. Ask him questions about it if you can.

- Consult with his doctor or pharmacist to see if he has a medical condition or a medication that may be the cause.

- If it is not dangerous or causing major upset, it may be best to accept the behaviour and/or ignore it.

- If the action is dangerous or causing major upset to you or others, try reassuring him, and gently redirect to a different activity.

- If the activity is a repetitive sound, like tapping his foot or humming, try to ignore it and/or put in earplugs.

- Answer the repetitive question in a calm way. Keep it brief and simple.

- Don't rush or come across as annoyed, as this may only cause him more concern and confusion.

- Don't point out he just asked the same question. It is likely he can't remember asking.

- Don't use a negative tone of voice to point out you already told him the answer. This may only upset him as he may genuinely not recall you answering him.

- He may feel unsure of himself due to memory loss and confusion.

- Use words of comfort. Try to be patient. He may just need to create a new positive emotional memory to recall your response.

- Use a loving touch, and look into his eyes. He may require extra reassurance. Try to connect with the feelings he has behind the actual question.

- Be aware of your tone of voice and how you use touch.

- Offer a distraction from the loop happening in his brain. Go for a walk or a relaxing drive. Look through photo albums, or watch a favourite TV program or movie.

- Give him a repetitive task, such as folding laundry, shredding papers, sanding wood blocks, winding balls of yarn, dusting, stacking magazines, polishing furniture/silverware, sorting, or sweeping.

- Make and have a snack together.

- Write the answer on a note. Use a white board to answer his questions, and leave it in a visible spot. Make flash cards with answers to the same questions.

- Try to give as little notice as possible of upcoming appointments or events. This may lessen the anxiety and repeated questioning.

18. Repetitive Sounds

Problem: Repetitive calling out, yelling, or moaning can be very disturbing to others. Stopping these behaviours can be very difficult. It is very common in late-stage dementia.

Solutions:

- Look into the reason why he is yelling/calling out.

- Offer reassurance as needed, including Therapeutic Reasoning®.

- Ask him if anything is wrong and if you can help.

- Speak to him with a calm and reassuring tone. Let him know he is safe.

- If he enjoys affection, offer a hug or a hand massage. Hold his hand for a few moments. This can be comforting and distracting.

- Offer a shoulder or back rub.

- Offer to sit with him, and watch TV or a movie, or do another pleasant activity, as he may be feeling alone and scared.

- Put on some of his favourite music, as this can also be distracting and comforting.

- Play old family home videos to see if that offers some comfort.

- Try taking him for a walk to get a change of scenery.

- Have a mental health professional assess to see if there is anything else that can be done.

19. Rummaging/Hoarding

Problem: Sometimes he will search through drawers and closets and also may like to collect objects. Sometimes things are pulled out and put into other, inappropriate, places such as in bags or boxes, making for a cluttered environment. Items then may become misplaced, causing more frustration (see: Hiding and Misplacing Objects). Hoarding may occur because of fear of not having enough of this one object or be due to an obsessive-compulsive disorder (OCD).

Solutions:

- For early stages, offer psychological support.

- Go slowly, and expect gradual changes.

- Treat him with respect and dignity.

- Avoid making negative, teasing, or sarcastic comments.

- Create one drawer or box full of items of interest. Items such as safe tools, photocopied photographs, keys, gloves, old watches, etc.

- To help reduce anxiety and frustration, offer to help him find what he is looking for. After a short while, redirect with another pleasurable activity.

- Reduce the number of things in his drawers, closets, and immediate environment. Remove things that may cause emotional upset or physical harm.

- If he likes to pack up his belongings in bags or suitcases, decide if you think this causes harm or not. If not, a harmless activity like this can keep him busy.

- If you notice he is hiding food items that will spoil, you may want to remove the items from easy access.

- If you must, go through his things and tidy when he is not around.

- If he appears to be in distress, help him look for what he is searching for, or offer a "break," a much-needed distraction.

- If anxiety is present for objects he no longer has, perhaps offer to take him out shopping for these items.

- Use a smart tracker device for items of importance that are often misplaced.

- Lock away valuable items.

20. Sexual Expression

Problem: Some people with dementia will demonstrate unwanted or inappropriate sexual expression or sex talk. They may expose themselves. It may be due to the inability to filter, or stop, these behaviours or thoughts, leading to some very unpleasant situations. Sexual expression can be verbal or physical.

Solutions:

- If he removes his clothing, find out if the behaviour is related to a nonsexual issue, such as needing to go to the toilet, pain/infection, uncomfortable clothing, or feeling hot.

- Don't scold or be judgmental.

- Validate his feelings. For example, "I know you are feeling frisky, but that will have to wait until a more appropriate time."

- Don't overreact to the sexual statements or requests. Calmly and quietly, tell him what he is saying or doing is not appreciated, and ask that it stop. Clarify what your role or task is. It is unlikely the behaviour will stop completely, but it may help. This is also known as "correction in the moment."

- Try saying to him, "Sorry, we don't talk like that around here."

- Avoid giggling or laughing at inappropriate remarks or behaviour.

- If he is inappropriately touching you or himself in public, try giving him something to hold, like a towel or article of clothing so his hands are full and he can't touch you or himself in private places.

- In some cases, you may be able to ignore the behaviour, requests, or statements.

- Work on making it difficult for the situation to repeat itself. For example, position yourself differently when providing personal-care tasks, wear different clothes, or distract with conversation, an object of interest, or singing.

- Try not to put yourself into a situation where you could be inappropriately groped, such as leaning over him.

- Ask him to do as much for himself as possible with respect to personal-care tasks. For example, hand him the cloth to wash his genitals, and keep privacy to a maximum.

- Encourage other family members to offer affection as appropriate.

- Privacy may need to be given for masturbation.

- If he is often removing his pants and inappropriately exposing himself, try providing him with clothes that are harder to remove, such as coveralls or special one-piece outfits.

- If you normally are intimate but are not feeling comfortable in the current moment, or if you feel you may need to use Therapeutic Reasoning®, you may want to state you love him, too, and will be sure you get together later on, but right now is not a good time.

- If he is making inappropriate sexual comments to family members or friends, you may want to inform them they need to be assertive by saying they do not like to be spoken to this way. They can also approach him using nicknames such as

"Buddy" or "Pal" to help establish a tone of friendship and to avoid close contact.

21. Sleep Problems

Problem: People living with dementia can have difficulty sleeping at night. Sometimes they sleep too much during the day. Sometimes they are up early or throughout the night. Perhaps they wander around the home, attempt to leave the premises, and/or make meals when no one is up to supervise them (see: Wandering; Wanting to "Go home").

Solutions:

- A sudden change in sleep habits could indicate a medical problem. Consider making a doctor's appointment.

- Talk to a pharmacist to see if his medications may be having an effect.

- The doctor may suggest some kind of sleep aid or sedating medication on a short-term basis. Use caution here, as some medications of this type can cause unwanted side effects such as increased risk for falls, daytime drowsiness, and increased confusion.

- Try keeping a consistent routine before bed.

- Be sure he does not go to sleep too early.

- Try adding Melatonin as a supplement before bed.

- Engage in a quiet activity before bed such as listening to relaxing music.

- Try warm milk with a cracker or cookie before bed.

- Offer a shoulder or back rub to help calm him before bed.

- Try giving him a 10-minute aromatherapy (fragranced or aromatic) hand massage.

- Encourage good sleep hygiene by avoiding caffeinated beverages later in the day.

- Discourage short naps after 3:00 p.m.

- Encourage plenty of exercise and fresh air during the day as much as possible.

- Increase exposure to daylight by having him sit near a window, or spend time outdoors.

- Put an alarm on the door so if it is opened, you will be alerted.

- Use a sensor mat on the bed to alert you when he gets up.

- Leave out a snack at night in case the person gets up and is hungry.

- Ensure there is a light on or use night-lights, so the washroom is easily found.

- Leave a urinal beside the bed so he doesn't have to get out of bed and make himself more awake.

- Change pillows, bedding, or nightclothes as necessary.

- You may need to enlist some help during the night if he continues to get up, such as night-duty shifts by other family members or even a paid home care worker.

22. Sundowning

Problem: Many people living with dementia experience an increase in restlessness, agitation, and confusion around the time the sun goes down. This could be due to many factors, including exhaustion, changes in lighting and shadows, or from past lifestyle habits and routines (coming home from work at that time). Do your best to become the detective to figure out why he may be behaving the way he is, and address it as best you can.

Solutions:

- Determine if the person has any unmet needs, such as needing to go to the bathroom, hunger, pain, or fatigue. Assist to make him feel more settled.

- If the reason is that he is hungry, but supper is not ready, offer him a snack every day around the same time just before you see his behaviour change.

- Perhaps serve dinner early, and offer a light snack before bedtime.

- If he is tired, encourage him to do a quiet and relaxing activity. To minimize the sundowning effect, encourage a rest earlier in the day (preferably before 3:00 pm).

- To minimize shadows and the effects of dusk, turn on lights and pull curtains before sunset.

- If he is restless, go for a walk with him, or find someone else to do this on a regular basis to build a routine.

- Provide calm reassurance according to his needs at all times.

- Gently reorient him to where he is and what time it is. If this doesn't work, then go into "his reality."

- Avoid saying, "No." Be creative in your responses, such as, "Sure, we can do that later or tomorrow."

- If medications have been prescribed to assist with Sundowning, be on the alert to see if they help, and be sure to combine with other environmental and behavioural solutions.

- Research suggests a low dose of Melatonin (a naturally occurring hormone) may induce sleepiness later in the evening.

- Rocking chairs are also good for this.

- Offer to go for a relaxing drive.

- Get outside and change the scenery.

- Play music, or put on a favourite program, and watch together.

- Offer a shoulder or back rub.

- Play some relaxing music.

- Try giving him a 10-minute aromatherapy (fragranced or aromatic) hand massage.
- Have a visitor come by to take him out in the mid-afternoon to help use up his energy.

- Reminisce about old times, or look through old photo albums together.

- Get him to help you make supper or bake.

23. Unsafe Driving

Problem: When a person has a diagnosis of dementia, it does not necessarily mean a doctor will take away his license to drive. However, when he is showing signs of unsafe driving practices, he should no longer have the privilege to drive. Getting lost and getting into accidents are sure signs it is time to hang up the keys. Sometimes the person does not see it that way, and he insists on driving anyway, posing a risk to himself as well as others. If you would not let your child or grandchildren go for a drive with him, then perhaps he is no longer a safe driver.

Solutions:

- Have a discussion about safety, and ask him to voluntarily give up his license.
- Consult with his family doctor about next steps.
- Validate his feelings. Show you're upset about all this, too, to help him feel comforted.
- Offer to drive him to get his groceries or get to appointments, etc.
- Consider hiring someone to drive him to appointments or take him out for drives if you aren't able.
- If he continues to drive even though his license has been taken away, to keep everyone safe, report this to the authorities, or have his doctor report him.
- If he continues to want to drive, disable the vehicle so it does not start (pull sparkplugs).

- Put a safety device over the steering wheel such as a Club.

- Hide the car keys or replace the car key with another to help keep the peace if he forgets he can't drive but feels more secure having a key set.

- Sell the car. "Out of sight; out of mind."

- When he asks for the car, say the car is "in the shop. We are waiting for a part to fix it." This technique, called "Therapeutic Reasoning®," is not harmful and will keep him and others safe.

- Put the car into storage, or park it somewhere different.

- Give him the number to a cab company to put in his wallet and on a sheet of paper where he can see it if need be.

24. Wandering

Problem: The person tends to walk, or pace, for long periods, seemingly without purpose. Maybe he is bored. Sometimes he is trying to find something familiar, or he is simply using pent-up energy to ease restlessness. Sometimes it can be healthy and safe. In some cases, wandering away may be a result of a goal or purpose to get somewhere else. It may no longer be a safe situation. Be on high alert when you notice wandering starting to happen.

Solutions:

- Enroll in the MedicAlert Safely Home program with the Alzheimer's Society. Receive an identification bracelet or necklace he can wear which can help get him back home.

- Look into using a GPS tracking device.

- Create identification cards, and ensure copies are in his wallet and coat/pants/shirt pockets at the beginning of each day. If he becomes lost, his name, address, and phone number are on the card, and he can be returned home safely.

- Ask him where he is going. Then ask him what he needs to do when he gets there. Alter your approach to best support him, according to his response.

- Try to determine if there is an unmet need, such as needing to use the toilet, hunger, pain, or discomfort.

- Take the person outside for a walk, or change his environment, as he may be wanting/trying to do this.

- Keep the person out of harm's way by making sure he is not going to trip or fall on something.

- Try using "child-safe" plastic doorknob covers to prevent him from leaving the house.

- Install a sliding door lock or chain link latch up high so it is not easily seen and is out of reach.

- Put a curtain or other soft barrier over the door so it is not easily recognized as a door. Alternatively, simply put a small towel (preferably the same colour as the door) over the doorknob.

- Use a door alarm, so if the door is opened, you will be alerted.

- He may follow or "shadow" you. Reassure him you love him and he is okay. Redirect him by suggesting an enjoyable and interesting activity.

- Regular exercise can help reduce restlessness.

- Let your neighbours know about his condition and your concerns, and give them a number where they can reach you or another family member if they notice him leaving on his own.

- Sometimes the person wants to leave or go out by himself, and this causes risks (see: Wants to "Go home").

25. Wants to "Go home"

Problem: People with late-stage dementia often fail to recognize their familiar surroundings, and want to "go home" or "leave" although they are, in fact, in their own home or in a family member's home. Sometimes it is difficult to convince the person he is at home. If he leaves and becomes lost, he is at risk by being exposed to the elements and/or other unsafe situations. Sometimes going home simply means feeling safe. It is always best to uncover the reason for his need to leave by asking him or by being a detective.

Solutions:

- Enroll in the MedicAlert Safely Home program with the Alzheimer's Society. Receive an identification bracelet or necklace he can wear which can help get him back home.

- Look into using a GPS tracker or other electronic locating device.

- Create identification cards and ensure copies are in his wallet and coat/pants/shirt pockets at the beginning of each day. If he becomes lost, his name, address, and phone number are on the card, and he can be returned home safely.

- When the person is expressing a need to leave, redirect him by asking him to help you out with something, or maybe offer a cup of coffee or a bite to eat first. The time it takes to do this may be just long enough for him to forget he wanted to leave in the first place.

- Ask him, "Where is your home?" Gather as much information as you can about the time of life, or era, he "thinks" he is in. Knowing *where* he is (in *his* mind) may help you understand the reasons for other behaviours.

- Have him talk about what he remembers about his home. Reminisce about the past and other fun topics. This conversation may help divert his need to "go home."

- Put a curtain or other soft barrier over the door so it is not easily recognized as a door. Alternatively, simply put a small towel (preferably the same colour as the door) over the doorknob to hide it.

- Try using "child-safe" plastic doorknob covers to prevent him from leaving the house.

- Install a sliding door lock or chain link latch up high so it is not easily seen and is out of reach.

- Use a door alarm, so if the door is opened, you will be alerted.

- Install sensors on the doors. A sensor can automatically alert you via text message, email, or even a phone call.

- Do not force him not to leave. Restraining him may only cause upset and may trigger physical aggression.

- Use validation for his feelings.

- Show with your body language you understand his situation by nodding your head in a positive way.

- Follow him only if it is safe to do so. Bring with you your coat, purse, and a cell phone.

- In some cases, it is best you do not follow him, as it may also put you at risk (exposure to the elements; trip or fall; he may get physical). Let someone else or the police find him instead.

- Offer a shoulder or back rub, as this may offer some comfort and reassurance.

- Play some of his favourite music.

- Go for a drive together.

- Say things that are reassuring, such as, "You are safe here," "I will help you get home later," "Tell me what happened," "You will feel better soon," "I can understand why you are upset," "I will look after this."

- Let your neighbours know about his condition and your concerns, and give them a number where they can reach you or another family member if they notice him leaving on his own.

- If you are driving your car and you find him, ask him where he is going. If he says, "I am going home," tell him with a smile, "Get in, I can take you there, as that's where I am going, too!"

- If he has left, and you cannot find him, let the police know, and they can help find him. Tell them what he was wearing, and have a photo ready to show them.

- Make distinguishing marks on the bottom of his shoes, and then photograph or photocopy the bottom of the shoes and the print they make. These sheets can be provided to police to help with a search for shoe prints.

- If you are unable to keep the person safe at home, you may need to consider having him move to a facility that can provide him with a specialized, higher level of supervision.

Challenging behaviours and other situations can arise at any stage of dementia. Being forewarned and forearmed can help make your role as wife and caregiver more manageable. Being aware of your own limits however, is very important. Sometimes the challenges cause so much stress and tension between the two of you, you may wonder if it has gone too far. In the next chapter, we will discuss abuse and neglect and what to watch for.

Exercise:

The main behaviour problems I have encountered so far are:

____

____

____

Some strategies that have worked are:

___

___

___

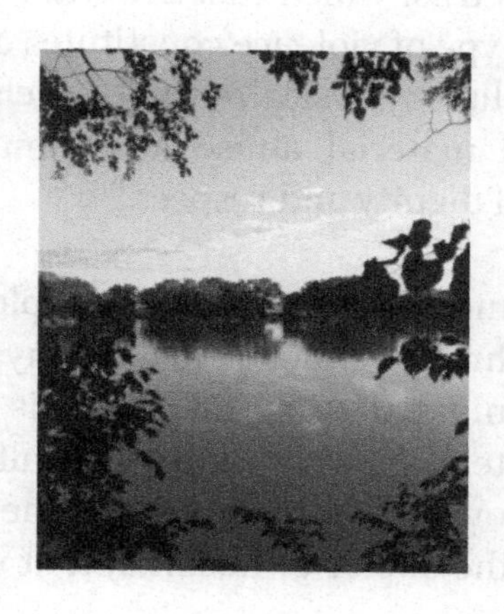

Chapter 15

Abuse and Neglect

Being thrust into the role of caregiver without any preparation is difficult under any circumstances.

— Carol Levine

One of the topics I am very passionate about is prevention of elder abuse. Social Work is dedicated to protecting those who are vulnerable. We see it in child welfare and intimate-partner violence. Social workers are trained to recognize and prevent abuse and neglect. Protection of older adults who are vulnerable, especially those who have dementia, is an important role of those who work in the field.

The definition of Elder Abuse, according to the World Health Organization (2014), is as follows:

> "Elder abuse is a single or repeated act, or lack of appropriate action, occurring within any relationship where there is an

> expectation of trust which causes harm or distress to an older person. This type of violence constitutes a violation of human rights and includes physical, sexual, psychological, emotional, financial and material abuse; abandonment; neglect; and serious loss of dignity and respect."

Sometimes it is important to educate people on what abuse is. Abuse is unwanted threats, either verbal or physical, that can cause someone to feel intimidated, or afraid. Abuse is what someone does to another person, intentionally or unintentionally. For example, if an older person tried to overdose on pills and his/her family member did not take him/her to the doctor or hospital, that would be considered abuse by neglect.

Caregiving can be a tough job. Tensions and stress may be high. Anger and agitation may result. Accusations and threats may occur. A shout, shove, or restraining technique is considered abusive. These behaviours may be demonstrated by not only the caregiver himself/herself but also by the person with dementia. Sometimes the abuse goes both ways. For the caregiver, his/her behaviour may feel justified, because he/she also feels "abused" by the person with dementia or other family members who live in the home. Lifelong relationship problems and patterns can also influence the type of abuse that occurs.

If or when this happens to you, please know there is help available. You can start by calling your local Alzheimer Society. Alternatively, you can talk to your physician. Refer back to Chapter 8 on How to Avoid Caregiver Burnout. Sometimes caregivers feel depressed or stressed to the point of exhaustion.

Abusive behaviours can happen at any time, especially when a person feels threatened. It can happen when a person feels like he/she is at the end of his/her rope. A well-cared-for caregiver has a better chance at reducing the occurrences of being abusive towards his/her loved one. Knowing the signs and symptoms of caregiver stress and burnout can help prevent any untoward events. Maltreatment of another person can happen in a progressive manner. Taking care of yourself and your loved one is vital to avoiding situations of abuse or neglect.

A person who has dementia will feel more safe and calm with a caregiver who is also feeling safe and calm. If you feel you are heading down that slippery slope of abusive-type behaviour, or if you are not sure, please contact your doctor or another health care professional for help. Check for local resources on "Elder Abuse." A therapist or counsellor can also help.

Getting help with identifying your stressors and speaking to someone about your concerns can help alleviate some of the tension and agitation you may be feeling which, in effect, can help improve your relationship with your husband. Reading through the information in this book will ultimately help you understand what you need to do in order to reduce the risks of inadvertently abusing or neglecting your husband. Your local Alzheimer's Society or Association can help you with this as well.

Exercise:

In terms of abuse and neglect, the most important thing for me to remember is:

____

____

____

Reference:

World Health Organization (2014). Elder Abuse Fact sheet No 357. Retrieved from: *www.who.int/mediacentre/factsheets/fs357/en/*

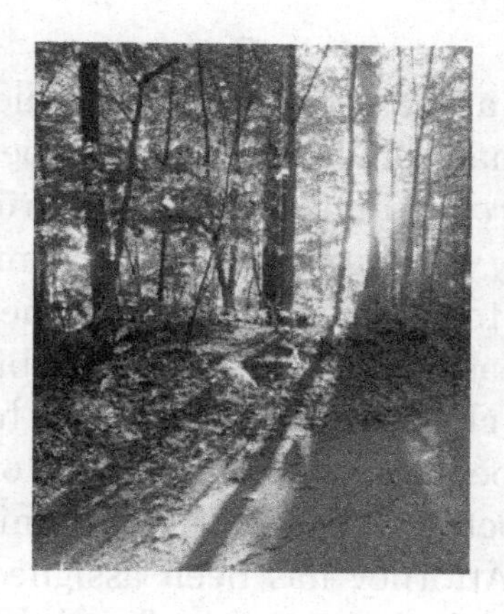

Chapter 16

Legal and Financial Preparedness

Knowledge is power.

— Francis Bacon

The topics of finances and legal matters can cause stress for caregiving wives. In many traditional households, the husband looks after the finances. If you always did the finances yourself, this may not be a stress area for you. In either case, I have found it helpful to go over some of the basic issues with respect to legal and financial issues. Some of this information you may already be aware of, and some of it may be new to you.

There are Elder Law Attorneys available if you need a lawyer to help draw up any legal documents. Your bank or credit union is also a good source for referrals to financial or legal professionals.

Power of Attorney

Power of Attorney is a legal document that indicates who you would like to act on your behalf should you no longer be able to manage your own *financial and property* matters. An enduring or durable Power of Attorney is highly recommended, as this means the appointed attorney will be able to act on your behalf in the unlikely event of an illness or injury such as dementia or traumatic brain injury. A trusted individual such as a child or other relative or friend is best for this job; however, some people choose a lawyer or other financial expert for this role. Contact a lawyer for more information. Once an enduring Power of Attorney has been assigned, a copy should be provided to the bank(s) where your husband does his business. You should also have notarized (authentic copy which is stamped or signed as such) copies on hand should the need arise.

Advanced Health Care Directive

An Advanced Health Care Directive (also known as a Living Will) comes into effect if you should not be able to make your own decisions in terms of health care. You can indicate in advance your wishes for treatment (such as Do Not Resuscitate). It will also indicate whom you wish to speak on your behalf in regard to medical decisions. This person is called your Health Care Proxy. In Ontario, the Health Care Proxy is designated Power of Attorney for Personal Care. Forms can be found on the Internet, or you can ask your doctor for more information.

Private Committeeship

If someone is no longer capable of looking after his or her own affairs due to illness or injury, and they require someone to help *make all decisions* for him or her, then a private committee may be appointed. A committee is a court-approved individual. Preferably, it is a close family member. Sometimes it is a person assigned by the court if no one else is available, willing, or able. It is a costly procedure, so not everyone chooses to go this route. The Public Guardian and Trustee office in your province has more information on this topic.

Will

A will or testament is a document that expresses your wishes as to what will happen to your possessions upon your death. This document is recommended for everyone, as it helps determine who will manage your estate after you are gone (Executor). It also allows you to specify how you want your assets distributed upon your death. Contact a lawyer to get more information on preparing a will. For more information on the role and duties of an Executor, search the Internet for "Role of executor in _________" (put your province or state in the blank).

Disability Tax Credit

The Disability Tax Credit is a non-refundable federal tax credit available to Canadians who have a severe or prolonged impairment in either physical or mental functioning. Prolonged impairment means the disability has lasted or will last at least 12 months, consecutively. The person who qualifies will have a "marked restriction" in their functioning in at least one of the following areas: speaking, hearing, walking, elimination (bowel or bladder functioning), feeding, dressing, performing the mental functions of everyday life, and ability to manage life-sustaining therapy/ treatment/medication to support vital functions. A qualified professional (doctor, psychologist, etc.) must complete the T2201 Disability Tax Credit Certificate. The application can go back up to 10 years prior.

At time of writing, the yearly tax savings amount was $7,766.00 for adults. The qualified professional can charge to have this form completed, and the charge can be applied as a medical expense on line 330 of the individual's tax return. The tax credits are transferable.

In terms of Mental Functions Necessary for Everyday Life, an example is given with respect to dementia:

A person exhibiting dementia, who coincidentally also suffers from diabetes and is unable to maintain his or her diabetes logbook or keep track of his or her glucose levels and insulin usage and who must rely on someone else to provide required care, may qualify for the DTC. In this case, the patient qualifies because his or her impairment affects both his and her adaptive functioning and memory to the extent that he or she is unable to live independently.

More information can be found on the Government of Canada, Canada Revenue Agency website, or by calling 1-866-741-0127. Your doctor should also be able to help you with this.

Primary Caregiver Tax Credit

In Manitoba, the Primary Caregiver Tax Credit recognizes the vital support caregivers provide to those needing care. It provides a refundable credit of up to $1,275.00 (at time of writing) per year to people who act as primary caregivers for spouses, relatives, neighbours, or friends who live at home in Manitoba. For this tax credit, people requiring care must be assessed at Level 2 or higher under the Manitoba Home Care Program guidelines. They are assessed based on the amount and type of care required for tasks like bathing, dressing, eating meals, mobility, and receiving medical care.

More information can be found on the Manitoba Government website, in the Manitoba Finance section, or by calling Manitoba Government Inquiry at 1-866-626-4862. Check for Caregiver Benefits in your province. For example, Nova Scotia has a Caregiver Benefit for those who qualify, at $400.00 per month (at time of writing).

Check out if there are any tax credits or other benefits available in your area. In Canada, contact the Canada Revenue Agency online. In the United States, try the Internal Revenue Service. Alternatively, ask an accountant if you qualify for any benefits. The Alzheimer Society or Association in your area may also be a good resource for information on this topic.

Joint Bank Accounts and Property Ownership

Some people decide to add a loved one or other trusted individual to their bank accounts and property titles. This is a way to safeguard their assets in the event they die or have some illness or injury that causes them to be incapable of managing their affairs. This makes it very easy for the other person to take over if something happens. Try to find out if you are on the accounts or house/property title. You will have to speak to the bank and/or a lawyer for any changes.

Legal Advice for Older Adults (65 Plus)

If there are complicated issues involving large sums of money, investments, property, businesses, or other matters that need to be resolved, you may want to seek a lawyer who specializes in *Elder Law*. You may also try searching the Internet for "legal guide seniors _________" (add your province or state in the blank) for more information on your rights.

Exercise:

Check off the following items *you have already* looked into or have done:

____ Power of Attorney
____ Advanced Health Care Directive/Power of Attorney Personal Care/Representation Agreement
____ Will
____ Joint Bank Accounts
____ Joint Title on House or Other Property if Owned
____ Disability Tax Credit

____ Tax Credits (e.g., Primary Caregiver Tax Credit, Manitoba)
____ Committeeship (May not be required)

I need to deal with the following issues:

____

____

____

The person or people who can help me with these issues are:

____

____

____

Conclusion

There are only four kinds of people in the world:
those who have been caregivers,
those who currently are caregivers,
those who will be caregivers,
and those who will need caregivers.

— Rosalynn Carter

I hope you have found this book helpful to you in your journey of caregiving a spouse who has a diagnosis of dementia or a related disorder. The information and lessons learned from the eight women who participated in the Wife Caregivers Project have proven to be invaluable to me, and I know if I should ever find myself in their position, I will feel more prepared to handle whatever may come my way.

I have learned about the commitment of marriage, the love shared between a husband and a wife, and the sacrifice and obligation that come with the vows of marriage. A dementia-affected long-term marriage built on memories, raising children, and ups-and-downs deserves an ending filled with care and love. It should be supported by not only the formal care system but also by informal supports.

Facing the "lion," the beastly parts of dementia, can be approached with confidence, courage, and commitment when they are better understood. Caregiving is enhanced when we have a better understanding of ourselves. This understanding can be gained from knowledge. I hope by reading this book (as well as many others), you will feel more empowered and prepared to manage the difficult and trying symptoms of dementia. You will also permit yourself to take care of your own needs.

My final hope for you is that you find others who are dealing with this issue, and you seek out the help that is right for you. You are not alone.

Exercise:

The best lesson I've learned about being a caregiver so far:

____

____

____

My personal goals in terms of caregiving for my husband are:

____

____

____

My next steps are:

____

____

____

Recommended Reading List

Boss, Pauline (2011). *Loving Someone Who Has Dementia: How to Find Hope While Coping with Stress and Grief.*

Boss, Pauline (2000). *Ambiguous Loss: Learning to Live with Unresolved Grief.*

Denholm, Diana B. (2012). *The Caregiving Wife's Handbook: Caring for Your Seriously Ill Husband, Caring for Yourself.*

Carpenter, Molly (2013). *Confidence to Care: A Resource for Family Caregivers Providing Alzheimer's Disease or Other Dementias Care at Home.*

Kubler-Ross, Elizabeth (2014). *On Death and Dying: What the Dying Have to Teach Doctors, Nurses, Clergy, and Their Own Families*. Scribner.

Mace, Nancy L. and Rabins, Peter V. (2011). *The 36-Hour Day: A Family Guide to Caring for People Who Have Alzheimer's Disease, Related Dementias, and Memory Loss.*

Marley, Marie and Daniel C. Potts (2015). *Finding Joy in Alzheimer's: New Hope for Caregivers.*

Marley, Marie (2011). *Come Back Early Today: A Memoir of Love, Alzheimer's, and Joy.*

Tyrell, Karen (2013). *Cracking the Dementia Code: Creative Solutions to Cope With Changed Behaviours.*

Resources and Organizations

Alzheimer's Association (USA)
225 North Michigan Ave., Floor 17, Chicago, IL 60601-7633
Tel: 312-335-8700/1-800-272-3900 (24-hour helpline)
TDD: 312-335-5886
Fax: 866-699-1246
Email: *info@alz.org*
Web: *www.alz.org*

Alzheimer Society of Canada
20 Eglinton Ave. W., Ste. 1600, Toronto, ON M4R 1K8
Tel: 416-488-8772
Toll-free: 1- 800-616-8816 (valid only in Canada)
Fax: 416-322-6656
Email: *info@alzheimer.ca*
Web: *www.alzheimer.ca*

Family Caregiver Alliance: National Center on Caregiving
Web: *www.caregiver.org*

The Mayo Clinic
Web: *www.mayoclinic.org/*

Well Spouse Association (USA)
63 West Main St., Suite H, Freehold, NJ 07728
Tel: 800-838-0879/732-577-8899
Fax: 732-577-8644
Email: *info@wellspouse.org*
Web: *www.wellspouse.org*

About the Author

Angela G. Gentile, B. S. W., M.S.W., R.S.W. is a specialist in aging who has more than 25 years of experience working with older adults and their families in a variety of capacities. She has worked in home care, geriatric mental health, long-term care, private practice, health care, and non-profit organizations.

In 1992, Angela obtained a Bachelor of Social Work degree from the University of Manitoba. In 2010, she obtained a Health Service Management Certificate from Red River College. In 2014, she obtained a Master of Social Work degree, with a Graduate Specialization in Aging, also from the University of Manitoba.

She is founder and manager of the LinkedIn Group, *Gerontology Professionals of Canada* and the *Aging Well for Women* Facebook page. She is a member of the Manitoba College of Social Workers.

Angela enjoys writing, traveling, photography, and exploring what it means to age well. She is a realistic optimist who lives in Winnipeg, Manitoba, with her husband and daughter. For more information on her books and services visit www.AngelaGGentile.com.

Made in United States
Orlando, FL
23 November 2024